# T O T A L
# Y O G A

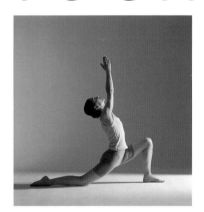

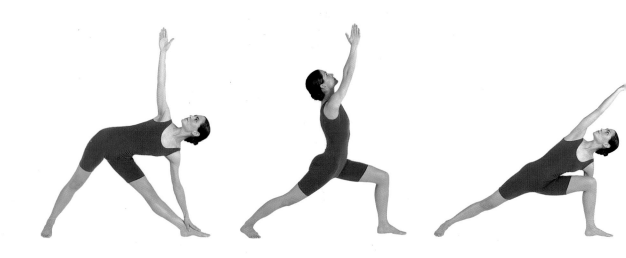

# TOTAL YOGA

*A step-by-step guide to yoga at home for everybody*

TARA FRASER

WATKINS PUBLISHING
LONDON

**For my mother Suzannah, who set me on this path.**

**Total Yoga**
Tara Fraser

Distributed in the USA and Canada by
Sterling Publishing Co., Inc.
387 Park Avenue South
New York, NY 10016-8810

This edition first published in the UK and USA in 2007 by
Watkins Publishing Limited
Sixth Floor
75 Wells Street
London W1T 3QH

A member of Osprey Group

Managing Editor: Judy Barratt
Editor: Kesta Desmond with Georgina Harris and Joanne Levêque
Managing Designer: Manisha Patel
Designer: Rachel Cross
Design Assistant: Simon Heard
Illustrator: Halli Verrinder
Model photography: Matthew Ward
Food photography: Sian Irvine

10 9

ISBN: 978-1-84483-409-9

Typeset in GillSans and Joanna MT
Color reproduction by Scanhouse, Malaysia
Printed in Singapore by Imago

Note on abbreviations
BCE (Before the Common Era) is the equivalent of BC.
CE (Common Era) is the equivalent of AD.

For information about custom editions, special sales, premium
and corporate purchases, please contact Sterling Special Sales
Department at 800-805-5489 or specialsales@sterlingpub.com.

"There is no trap like illusion, no greater strength than yoga, no greater friend than knowledge, no greater enemy than pride."

*Gheranda Samhita*

# contents

# how to use this book

This book describes in simple terms the basics of Hatha yoga (see page 15). If you are a total beginner, you can use the step-by-step explanations and photographs in chapters 4 and 5 to start practising yoga for the first time. If you are already attending a yoga class, this book will provide you with background knowledge, and guidance on how to do the postures at home (self-practice).

There are eight chapters: the first gives general background information on the history and theory of yoga and why it remains as relevant to our lives today as it was to the ancient sages. Yoga can be applied to all aspects of our lives – including what we eat. This, as well as drinking and fasting, is explored in Chapter 2. Chapter 3 looks at the practice of posture, or *asana*: how to find a style of yoga and a class that's right for you, and how to start yoga by yourself at home. Chapters 4 and 5 are step-by-step guides to postures and sequences; and chapters 6 and 7 introduce breathing and meditation techniques. Chapter 8 is a guide to the yoga postures that you can practise with a friend or partner.

Please read each chapter from beginning to end before attempting any of the fasts, postures, sequences, or meditation and breathing exercises. This will give you all the background and safety information you need. When you are trying out postures for the first time it may be helpful to have a partner read the instructions aloud to you. At

least look at both the instructions and photographs before starting –
the photographs alone will not always give you enough information
to get safely into a pose and gain maximum benefit from it.

I have chosen photographs that show the postures as clearly as
possible. All the models have been practising yoga for many years –
so don't despair if you don't look exactly like them! Concentrate on
how a posture feels rather than what it looks like. Go to a teacher
as often as you can to check your technique and gain inspiration.

Whether you are a complete beginner or are already attending
classes, I hope this book will encourage, inspire and challenge you –
enjoy your practice.

---

### SYMBOLS USED IN THIS BOOK

An easier modification of a posture to be used if you are a beginner, if you are
having difficulty in a pose or if you simply want a softer yoga practice.

A more physically demanding way of doing a posture that is suitable if you are
familiar with the posture or want to try a stronger practice.

Ideas, tips and comments that will help you in a posture.

A caution about when to avoid a posture or what to do if it causes you pain
or discomfort.

# introduction

I did my first ever yoga class as a small child, alongside my mother, in London in the 1970s. I can clearly remember the lovely sensation of practising deep backbends in that sunny room, and of finding new ways to move and stretch. Many years later, having suffered a nasty back injury, I returned to yoga as a way to heal myself where painkillers and conventional therapies had failed. This time, rather than deep backbends, I was doing very simple breathing exercises to relieve the pain. My teacher and I sat back-to-back and breathed together. I began to notice how tense I was, how my breathing was shallow and apologetic. I slowly regained sensation in my body – it was like thawing out after years of being frozen. Through gentle, persistent practice my back felt better. And, in the process, I learned about my body and the connections between body, breath and mind.

When I began to teach yoga, a whole new world opened up to me. It was amazing to watch hundreds of different bodies try out the postures and breathing exercises. I came to appreciate that yoga is an individual path for everyone who undertakes it – no two people are the same and no two yoga practices are alike.

I carried on learning from both my teachers and my students. My personal practice was strong and athletic. When I became pregnant I enjoyed and learned a great deal from specialized antenatal classes. Then, after the birth of my son, I began to study with a

Viniyoga teacher whose soft and gentle approach was astonishingly effective. I went back to working with stillness, breath and focus, with less concern for the athletic postures that I was now (as a mother) simply too exhausted to do. Once again, I realized the importance of fitting yoga to my life, body and mental state.

Later still, the philosophy of yoga became my chief fascination and, finally, I felt ready to apply its principles to my life. The evolution of my spiritual responses has surprised me at times (having been a natural sceptic and not inclined toward the "mystical" areas of life). But here I am embarking on a fully fledged spiritual practice.

In writing this book I hope that I have imparted some of my enthusiasm, as well as helpful guidelines, for your practice. Yoga is a wonderful tool for everybody: young or old; healthy or sick; man, woman or child. Whether you begin with the aim of becoming spiritually enlightened or just stretching your legs is not important. The point is to begin and to see where the journey takes you.

*Tara Fraser*

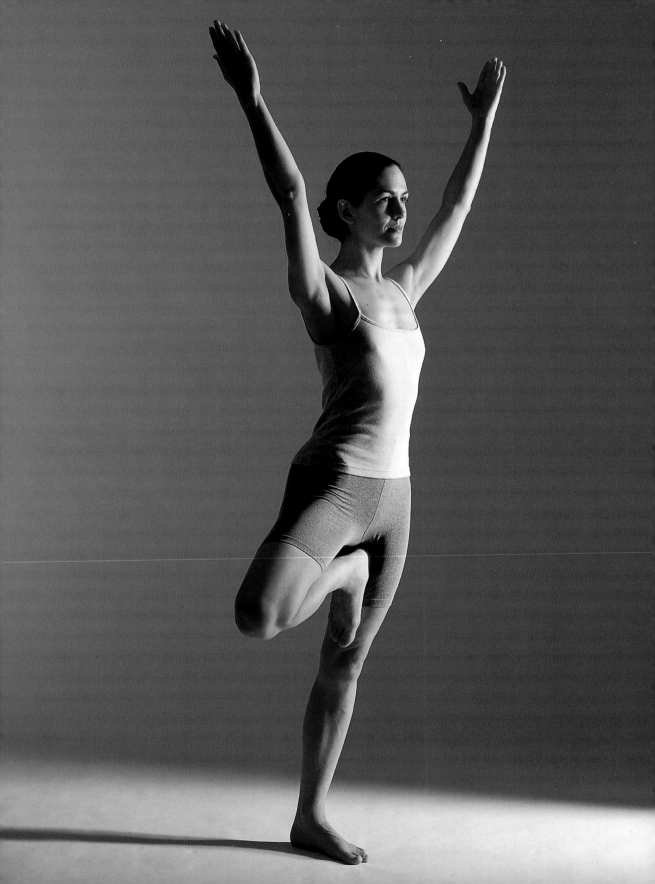

# the art of union

Yoga, the union of our physical, mental and spiritual selves, is far more than a form of exercise — it is a way of life. Although many of us gain our first introduction to yoga by going to classes which help to relax or tone our bodies, we soon find that yoga also encourages us to focus our minds and become more aware of the internal flow of energy.

The holistic doctrines of yoga are the result of thousands of years of experimentation and observation by great sages, enlightened gurus and ordinary people like you and me.

This chapter looks at the principles and philosophy of yoga as described in the key texts; the yogic view of the subtle anatomy; and the relevance of yoga in the contemporary West.

# what is yoga?

Yoga is a branch of Indian philosophy. The Sanskrit word "yoga" has many meanings among which is to "yoke" or "unite", referring to the union of the individual self with the universal consciousness (or "Absolute"). But yoga also describes the union of the physical body with the mind and spirit as a method of transcending the limitations of the ego and reaching enlightenment.

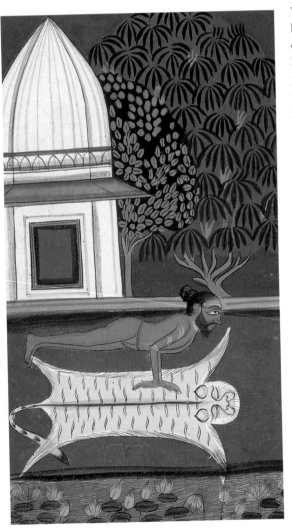

Yoga has existed in some form for thousands of years. Its history, which can be traced back to the time of the Vedic culture – around 2800BCE – is closely entwined with the Hindu religion (Vedic philosophy was also the starting point of Hinduism). Yoga, which is closely associated with Hinduism and other traditions including Buddhism, Jainism and Tantra, is best described as a spiritual rather than a religious practice. This means that anyone can practise yoga: it can be incorporated into a religious belief or it can be practised alone as a form of secular spirituality. Yoga provides humankind not only with a spiritual path but also with a method for "right living"; a set of moral, ethical and practical guidelines that help you to live a balanced and healthy life.

The earliest references to yoga come from sculptures and carvings dating back as far as 2800BCE, that were found in the Indus Valley (in modern Pakistan). These artefacts were made by the Vedic people, a Sanskrit-speaking race, whose scriptures – the *Vedas* – are among the oldest in the world. The *Vedas* gave rise to *Vedanta* – a huge and varied collection of texts, among which are the *Upanishads* and the *Bhagavad Gita* (see page 17). These texts – and others – form the basis of Hindu philosophy and yogic literature.

There are several different paths of yoga and each one approaches the ultimate goal of self-realization by a different route. Although these paths may seem disparate,

*This 18th-century Indian painting shows a yogi performing asana (posture) practice. Posture is just one way of practising yoga. Other ways include study, meditation, prayer, selfless action and mantra.*

and sometimes contradictory, they are all based on the premise that human beings can, through their own actions, become one with the Absolute. This concept is also known as enlightenment, self-realization, union of the individual self with the universal self, *Atman* with *Brahman* or *Prakriti* with *Purusha*.

The six main paths of yoga are described below. Within each path, there are separate branches or styles. See pages 44–5 for the different styles of Hatha yoga.

## Jnana yoga

This is the path of wisdom and is most suited to people with an intellectual temperament. The practitioner seeks to find his or her true self by the pursuit of knowledge – ignorance is seen as the obstacle to enlightenment. The main practices of Jnana yoga are study and meditation.

## Bhakti yoga

This is the path of devotion and is most suited to people who are attracted to prayer. The principle of Bhakti yoga is that we become as the things that we love and worship. By worshipping a god or guru who has achieved enlightenment we can achieve it ourselves.

## Karma yoga

This is the path in which the practitioner devotes his or her life to selfless action. The emphasis is not so much upon the magnitude of the action as on its motive. For example, someone who completes an action with love is practising Karma yoga, whereas someone who is driven by reward is not.

## Mantra yoga

This is the path of sacred sound. Self-realization comes from repetition – silently or aloud – of sacred sounds, phrases or words known as mantras.

The yogi focuses on the mantra to the exclusion of all else. The most sacred yoga mantra is the single syllable "OM" (see page 121).

## Raja yoga

Raja means "Royal". This is an eight-step path to enlightenment. The steps include the practice of posture, breath control, meditation and withdrawal of the senses. This eight-step path is defined in detail in a yoga text called the *Yoga Sutras* (see pages 18–19).

## Hatha yoga

This is the path of physical control and is properly regarded as a preparation for the pursuit of Raja yoga (for which physical strength and breath control are needed). Hatha yoga is the type of yoga that is most widely practised in the West, and the type that is covered in this book – when Westerners refer to "yoga", they usually mean Hatha yoga.

The word "Hatha" means "forceful". Although this may not be a word that you immediately associate with yoga, the practices of Hatha yoga can indeed be powerful. The individual syllables "Ha", meaning "sun", and "tha", meaning "moon", unite in the word "Hatha", suggesting the union of opposites. The harmonizing of opposing forces is a key aspect of yoga – hot energy is united with cool energy, strong with soft, and masculine with feminine.

Hatha yoga employs a combination of physical postures, breathing exercises, cleansing processes and mindful awareness of the physical and subtle bodies (see page 21) to prepare for contemplation and meditation.

# the texts of yoga

Hatha yoga is principally an oral tradition that has been passed down from teacher to student. But much of yoga's wisdom has also been written down in the form of verses, aphorisms and practical guides. As a result, there is a wealth of texts to offer inspiration and guidance and which provide an excellent source of material for the in-depth study of yoga. These texts are part of a huge and complex body of work known collectively as *Vedanta*. It is thought that the published works of yoga (of which there are many) represent a fraction of the manuscript material existing in the private libraries of India.

For students of yoga in the West, it is often surprising and encouraging to find out just how direct, fresh and relevant the texts of yoga are to their own practice. While some texts are cryptic (deliberately so) and need to be decoded by a teacher, others seem to jump off the page and speak straight to the reader. For example, the *Hathayoga Pradipika* describes the techniques for postures such as *padmasana* (lotus pose), *gomukhasana* (cow-face pose) and *savasana* (corpse pose) almost exactly as you will learn them in a class or read in Chapter 4. Even the more metaphysical texts such as the *Amritabindu Upanishad* contain direct and practical advice ("Mastery of the mind leads to wisdom. Practice meditation. Stop all vain talk.") and the *Bhagavad Gita* asserts that yoga is for everyone – even you!

Most of the principal texts of yoga were originally written in the archaic Indian language of Sanskrit. (For contemporary readers, excellent translations with detailed commentaries are now available all over the world.) Some texts are written in the form of aphorisms or as dialogues between teacher and pupil; some are practical treatises; and others are epic poems or exquisite hymn-like verses. Each one throws its unique light on the practice of yoga. They do not all agree on the detail or even on the main

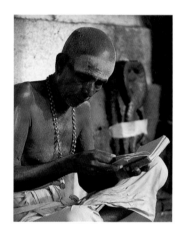

*Yoga posture practice can be complemented by reading and learning about the philosophy of yoga.*

points of yoga practice or philosophy. This is not surprising given the antiquity and diversity of the tradition of yoga and the fact that India is an enormous country. Before the age of motorized transport and mass communication, individual pockets of tradition developed in different areas from the teachings of each guru. To this day, no comprehensive study of the entire body of yogic writings has been carried out.

The key text upon which modern Hatha yoga (see page 15) is based is the *Yoga Sutras* (see pages 18–19). Other important texts are as follows.

### Goraksha Paddhati

This work contains 202 verses that describe a six-step path for yogis to follow: posture, breath control, sense withdrawal, concentration, meditation and ecstasy (similar to the eight-step path in the *Yoga Sutras*). This text also describes the energy centres of the body, and stresses the importance of the repetition of "OM" (see page 121).

### Hathayoga Pradipika

The title of this 14th-century manual is translated as "light on Hatha yoga". The *Hathayoga Pradipika* unites the physical practice of Hatha yoga with the spiritual aims of

Raja yoga (see page 15). The work includes descriptions of the seals and locks (*bandha*) that arouse *kundalini* energy (see page 23), and eight different types of breath control.

## Gheranda Samhita

Gheranda's "compendium" was written in the late 17th century and describes more than 30 postures, 21 cleansing techniques and 25 "seals" or *mudras* (see page 119). It also lists the types of food that should be eaten and offers advice on eating habits: "Half the stomach should be filled with food, one quarter with water, and one quarter should be kept empty for *pranayama* [breath control]."

## Bhagavad Gita

Meaning the "song of the blessed one", the *Bhagavad Gita* is part of the *Mahabharata*, the great Hindu epic poem. The author Vyasa is said to have written the text during the 6th century BCE. It takes the form of a dialogue between prince Arjuna, the hero, and the Hindu god Krishna. The first six chapters describe the path of Karma yoga, the

next six describe Bhakti yoga and the last six describe Jnana yoga (see page 15). The entire work also expounds the ideal of Purnayoga – a synthesis of all three types.

## Upanishads

The word *upanishad* means "to sit down next to" and describes how a student sits down next to a guru in order to learn. The *Upanishads* consist of more than 200 texts that are believed to contain the ultimate truth. Of these 200, 21 are "Yoga-*Upanishads*", but all are worthy of study in relation to yoga. The *Upanishads* were written over a huge span of time: some are more than 3,000 years old, others were written in the 20th century. Mostly metaphysical rather than practical in content, they include the concepts of reincarnation, karma and yoga as a route to the liberation of the self (breaking the cycle of death and rebirth).

*The Mahabharata is an ancient Hindu epic that contains the Bhagavad Gita, which expounds the philosophy of yoga. The detail here shows a 16th-century illustrated page with Sanskrit text.*

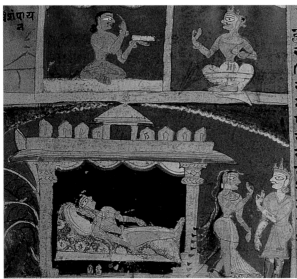

# Patanjali's *Yoga Sutras*

Probably the single most influential text on yoga, the *Yoga Sutras* are thought to have been written between 200BCE and 200CE. Despite the importance of this work, its author Patanjali remains an enigma – almost nothing is known about his life. In the *Sutras*, Patanjali details eight steps or "limbs" for the practice of Raja yoga (see page 15). The third and fourth limbs – posture (*asana*) and breath control (*pranayama*) – form the basis of modern yoga practice.

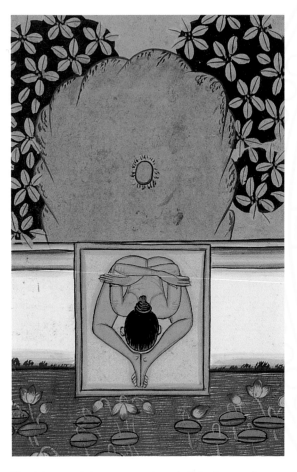

The 18th-century Indian manuscript from which this figure is taken illustrates a yogi in a seated pose. Patanjali lists posture practice (asana) as the third limb of Raja yoga.

Patanjali's Yoga Sutras consist of 195 aphorisms – condensed nuggets of wisdom that are traditionally elucidated by a teacher (guru). The word sutra means "thread", from which we get the English word "suture" meaning "to stitch". The Sutras thread together a series of philosophical concepts that, in practice, provide the route to self-realization. By using a terse writing style, Patanjali preserved both the essence of meaning in the Sutras and the student–teacher tradition. The Sutras are concise enough to be easily memorized, recited or chanted (the traditional way of learning them), and profound enough to support hours of discussion with a teacher. The precise meaning of each Sutra is a matter of interpretation and can be tailored to the needs of individual students. A teacher will guide students toward the aspect of each Sutra that they need to consider.

The Sutras are divided into four chapters. Patanjali is said to have written each chapter specifically for one of four disciples. Since each disciple had a different temperament and aptitude, the chapters vary in their approach. The essence of each of the four chapters has been described very simply as contemplation, method, exceptional faculties and serenity. Each chapter can be read as a complete teaching in itself, as well as a part of the Sutras as a whole.

The first chapter defines yoga and lists the difficulties we may encounter in the practice of yoga and how to overcome them. Patanjali defines yoga as "the ability to direct and sustain mental activity without distraction" (*yogah citta-vrtti-nirodhah*).

## THE EIGHT LIMBS OF YOGA

In the second chapter of the *Yoga Sutras* (*Sutra* II.29), Patanjali sets out eight limbs of yoga that practitioners should follow in order to develop the level of discernment and clarity of perception necessary to achieve a state of enlightenment. The eight limbs are as follows:

1. *Yama*: social conduct, which comprises non-violence (*ahimsa*), truthfulness (*satya*), non-stealing (*asteya*), moderation in sex and in all things (*brahmacarya*) and non-greed (*aparigraha*).
2. *Niyama*: individual conduct, which comprises purity or cleanliness (*sauca*), contentment (*santosa*), austerity (*tapas*), the study of texts (*svadhyaya*) and awareness of and devotion to the divine (*Isvarapranidhana*).
3. *Asana*: posture (see chapters 3–5).
4. *Pranayama*: breath control (see Chapter 6).
5. *Pratyahara*: sense withdrawal, which means turning the senses away from the external social and physical world to the internal mental, intellectual and spiritual world. This facilitates concentration and meditation.
6. *Dharana*: concentration.
7. *Dhyana*: meditation (see Chapter 7).

8. *Samadhi*: the superconscious state leading to self-realization that is the ultimate purpose of yoga.

The state of *samadhi* itself is an intense form of concentration that arises from the seventh limb, *dhyana*. The mind becomes so clearly focused on a single point that the practitioner experiences absolute unity between himself and the focus of his concentration. This blissful state may not be held for long at first, but can, with regular practice, be sustained, developed and entered at will.

Although the *Yoga Sutras* were written thousands of years ago, the eight limbs remain a useful template for us to follow today. Patanjali's eight limbs need not be practised in numerical order. Neither is it necessary to complete one step in order to progress to the next. Many of us start with the practice of posture, which leads us to breath control and concentration. These, in turn, may lead us into a greater awareness of how we conduct ourselves, both personally and socially. In this way, we can be working on *yama*, *niyama*, *asana*, *pranayama* and *dhyana* all at once or individually. Patanjali's eight limbs are intertwining threads or paths leading to the ultimate goal of *samadhi*.

The second chapter explains the qualities needed to concentrate the mind and how to attain these qualities. The third chapter describes the extraordinary capacity of the mind when free from distractions; and the fourth discusses the possibilities for a person with a superbly concentrated mind.

### Obstacles to yoga practice

The *Sutras* also list nine obstacles (*antaraya*), which have commonly hampered or frustrated people's practice of yoga and which apply to us as much today as they did to the yogis of Patanjali's time. The obstacles are sickness, lack of mental effort, self-doubt, inattention, laziness or fatigue, over-indulgence or sensuality, false knowledge and misunderstanding, lack of concentration, and lack of perseverance.

People who encounter these obstacles may suffer pain, despair or depression, and unsteadiness in body or breathing. Patanjali offers practical, physical solutions for overcoming these obstacles (and the symptoms they give rise to): *asana* for cultivating bodily strength and vitality and *pranayama* to help still the mind.

# prana and the subtle body

The yogic concept of energy is known as *prana*, a force that operates both within our physical bodies and in the world around us. The complexity of this concept is notorious, leading the great teacher B.K.S. Iyengar to comment, "It is as difficult to explain *prana* as it is to explain god." Different schools of yoga have found various ways to describe in detail the nature of *prana*. They all agree that it is a kind of "life-force", a universal flow of energy that gives us — and other living things — the spark of life.

The idea that there is an intangible life-force present in the universe is recognized by a variety of cultures. The Chinese call this life-force *chi* and chart its flow through channels called meridians (similar to the Indian *nadis*; see page 23). The Japanese call it *ki* and say that it resides in the abdomen. Modern science has not "discovered" *prana* yet, but people who practise yoga become strongly aware of its nature. As more research into traditional therapies and medicines is carried out in the West, our acceptance of and respect for these older theories deepen.

To develop our understanding of *prana* we can compare it to electric current. Like *prana*, electricity existed in the world before mankind discovered it; we cannot see, smell or touch it. Yet electricity influences our daily lives in various forms, from lightening bolts and static electricity to computers and electric lights. *Prana* is present both in our bodies and in the external world. It exists in all life forms, but also in the elements — water, air, earth and fire. We can absorb *prana* by eating, drinking and breathing and we can also obtain it from sunshine, wind and rain. Some schools of yoga maintain that there is a finite amount of *prana* in the body which we only need to circulate effectively. All agree that *prana* is the vital energy that sustains life. The *Kaushitaki Upanishad* explains, "Life is

*Prana is a subtle form of energy that circulates around the body in channels known as nadis. It exists outside the body too — air, sunlight, water and trees are all strongly charged with prana.*

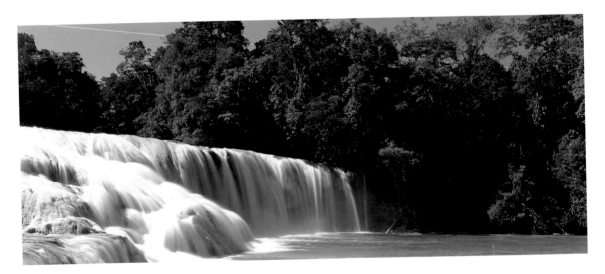

prana, prana is life. So long as prana remains in this body, there is life." The beautiful text of the *Prashna Upanishad* gives another description, "Everything rests in prana, as the spokes rest in the hub of a wheel."

## The subtle body
According to yogic theory, human beings exist in both a physical and a subtle form. The subtle body can be divided into four distinct but connecting layers or "sheaths". The first layer is made up of networks of channels (*nadis*) through which *prana* flows, and it is therefore called the *pranic sheath* (*pranamaya kosha*). The second layer is the mental sheath (*manomaya kosha*), which is our subconscious mind; the third is the intellectual sheath (*vij-nanamaya kosha*), which corresponds to both the conscious, controlling mind and the ego. Finally, at the core of the being is the bliss sheath (*anandamaya kosha*), which contains the seed of the true self (*bindu*). Yoga views all the sheaths as "temporary bodies" which can be cast off like clothes when worn out, so the self can be reincarnated time and again until this cycle is transcended by enlightenment.

## The subtle anatomy
The subtle body has its own "anatomy" distinct from but relating to that of the physical body. A central channel or *nadi* running along the midline of the body is known as *sushumna*. Energy centres called *chakras* (see pages 24–7) are located along this central channel and at its base lies

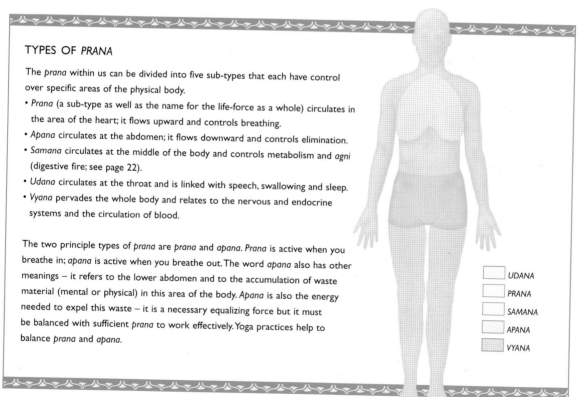

## TYPES OF *PRANA*

The *prana* within us can be divided into five sub-types that each have control over specific areas of the physical body.
• *Prana* (a sub-type as well as the name for the life-force as a whole) circulates in the area of the heart; it flows upward and controls breathing.
• *Apana* circulates at the abdomen; it flows downward and controls elimination.
• *Samana* circulates at the middle of the body and controls metabolism and *agni* (digestive fire; see page 22).
• *Udana* circulates at the throat and is linked with speech, swallowing and sleep.
• *Vyana* pervades the whole body and relates to the nervous and endocrine systems and the circulation of blood.

The two principle types of *prana* are prana and apana. Prana is active when you breathe in; *apana* is active when you breathe out. The word *apana* also has other meanings – it refers to the lower abdomen and to the accumulation of waste material (mental or physical) in this area of the body. Apana is also the energy needed to expel this waste – it is a necessary equalizing force but it must be balanced with sufficient prana to work effectively. Yoga practices help to balance prana and apana.

UDANA
PRANA
SAMANA
APANA
VYANA

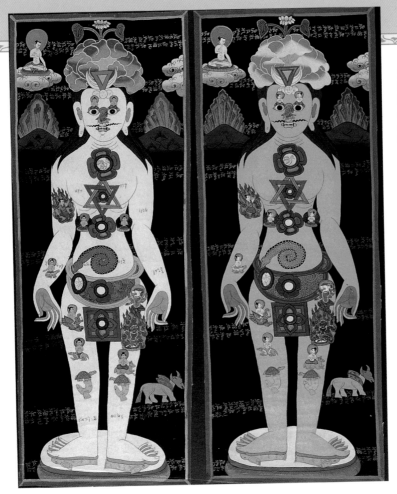

These 18th-century paintings of Nepalese figures show not only the chakras but also kundalini or serpent power. The coiled serpent in the abdomen symbolizes a form of energy that can be encouraged by yoga practice to rise up the central nadi.

power a machine efficiently, a body depleted of *prana* is weak and vulnerable to illness and disease. When the *nadis* are blocked, the flow of *prana* is impeded and this has a detrimental effect on our health. The balance and flow of *prana* can be upset by a multitude of things including our state of mind, and our past actions and current preoccupations. Eating a poor diet, drinking too much alcohol, smoking, leading a sedentary lifestyle and getting insufficient sleep will have a detrimental effect on the flow of *prana* and can result in tiredness, listlessness, depression and illness.

If we can encourage *prana* to flow freely we become stronger and more healthy. Applying the principles of *yama* and *niyama* (see page 19) to daily life can help to make positive changes and free blockages in the subtle body. On a physical level yoga prescribes *asana* (postures), *pranayama* (breath control), and *kriya* (cleansing exercises) as ways of clearing the *nadis* and positively influencing the flow of *prana*.

*Kriyas* are very strong cleansing practices for the physical and subtle bodies which produce profound results. Like all yoga practices they must be tailored to the individual's needs and are best learned from a teacher. Two *kriyas* are described in detail on pages 110 and 122 — *kapalabhati* and *trataka*, both of which are comparatively simple and mild, although very effective.

kundalini — a type of latent energy (see box opposite). *Agni* is the name given to the "digestive fire" located in the area of the navel. The flame of *agni* burns the waste matter that it encounters, thus purifying the body and clearing the path for a balanced flow of *prana*. This is why inverted postures, such as headstand (see pages 84–5), are important in yoga — they direct *agni* toward the abdomen and burn or neutralize waste known as *apana* (see page 21).

## Prana and health

Our health is directly affected by the flow of *prana* in the physical and subtle bodies. Just as a low battery will not

## NADIS AND *KUNDALINI*

*Nadis* are the channels throughout the *pranamaya kosha* (see page 21) along which *prana* flows. There are said to be 72,000 *nadis*, many of which are named. Three are of particular importance: *sushumna nadi*, *ida nadi* and *pingala nadi*. *Sushumna nadi* starts at the very base of the body at *muladhara chakra* (see page 25) and then rises in a straight line toward the crown of the head – the same path as the spinal cord in the physical body. Yoga practices will eventually encourage *prana* into this central channel. *Sushumna* is the perfect path for *prana* because *prana*'s effects can spread from here throughout the body without any vital energy being lost or dissipated.

On either side of *sushumna* are *ida* and *pingala nadis*. They spiral like a double helix around *sushumna* and exit at the nostrils. *Ida nadi* starts on the left side of *sushumna* and exits at the left nostril; *pingala nadi* starts on the right side of *sushumna* and exits at the right nostril.

Both *ida* and *pingala* have specific and opposite characters. *Ida nadi* is associated with female qualities and the cool energy of the moon – it corresponds to the part of the nervous system in the physical body that controls our restful state. *Pingala nadi* is associated with male qualities and the hot energy of the sun – it corresponds to the part of the nervous system in the physical body that controls our alert state. One result of alternate nostril breathing (see page 112) is the

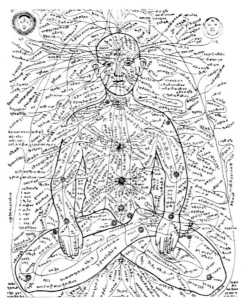

*There are thousands of nadis in the subtle body. The most important nadis are* sushumna, *and* ida *and* pingala, *which each spiral around* sushumna.

balancing of the flow of *prana* through *ida* and *pingala*.

At the bottom of *sushumna nadi* lies *kundalini* – the name given to a type of dormant female energy. *Kundalini* is symbolized as a sleeping serpent coiled three and a half times round the base of *sushumna* with her mouth covering the entrance to the *nadi*. Yoga practice can rouse this serpent and encourage it to rise up *sushumna* through the *chakras* (see page 25) toward the crown *chakra* – *sahasrara*.

As *kundalini* passes each *chakra*, a different state of conciousness is experienced. When *kundalini* reaches the crown *chakra*, a person is said to have reached *samadhi*: the ultimate stage of meditation when our true self can be realized beyond boundaries of mind, body and ego.

On its journey up toward the crown *chakra*, *kundalini* energy may encounter blockages known as *granthis*. These act as safety barriers to stop *kundalini* rising too fast or uncontrollably, which may result in physical or mental breakdown. The processes of Hatha yoga prepare the physical and mental body by gently freeing these blockages to enable *kundalini* to rise steadily to her goal.

The concepts of *nadis* and *kundalini* are common to the yoga tradition as a whole. If the emphasis in yoga practice is primarily on the raising of *kundalini* energy, then this form of yoga may be described as *Kundalini* yoga.

# the body's energy centres

At specific points along the midline of the body there are energy centres known as *chakras*. Each *chakra*, depicted in the shape of a lotus flower, has its own particular set of characteristics. The *chakras* are also associated with particular animals, gods and goddesses, and areas of influence. Yoga helps to develop awareness of the *chakras* and encourages energy flow toward them.

Like *prana* and *nadis* (see pages 20–23), *chakras* cannot be easily reconciled with a Western understanding of anatomy and physiology. They exist in the subtle body (see page 21) but they also have close links with the physical body and coincide with the position of nerve plexuses (networks) along the spinal cord. In the subtle body, they are located at the points where the three principle *nadis* – *pingala*, *ida* and *sushumna* – intersect.

## Wheels of light

The word "*chakra*" means wheel. At the points where the *chakras* occur, the *prana* flowing through the *nadis* spins to form brightly shining circles or "wheels of light". Most people's *chakras* are said to exist as small faint circles, whereas the *chakras* of a yoga practitioner should be bright and vibrant. Although the *chakras* are part of the subtle anatomy and cannot be seen by the eye, you may become highly sensitive to their energy through the practice of yoga. In fact, experience of the *chakras* through your own yoga practice is probably the best route to truly understanding them.

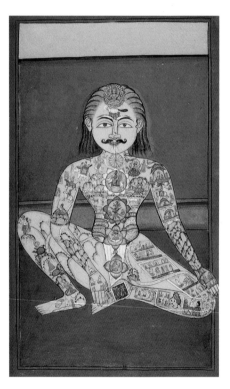

This 18th-century painting of a Nepalese yogi shows how the chakras follow a line along the centre of the body starting at the perineum and finishing at the crown of the head.

## Characteristics of the *chakras*

Each *chakra* has its own unique properties and is associated with a particular part of the body (and network of nerves), a shape, an element, a colour, a mantra on the petals, a "seed" (*bija*) mantra, and a *siddhi* (special power). Even the number and colour of petals in the symbolic lotus flower is specific to the *chakra*. In the Hindu yoga tradition, deities are associated with each *chakra*. Some other traditions attribute gem stones, astrological signs and plants to the *chakras*.

The precise nature and number of the *chakras* varies depending on the particular text or tradition that you consult. In Tibetan Buddhism, for example, there are only five *chakras*. Other yoga texts mention 12 or more *chakras* represented by lotus flowers with millions or even billions of petals. However, the majority of yoga traditions favour the view that there are six *chakras* plus *sahasrara* at the top of the head (although we refer to *sahasrara* as a *chakra*, strictly speaking it is the point at or above the crown of the head at which we transcend bodily existence).

## How yoga practice influences the chakras

When you perform the strong bending and twisting postures in yoga you free up prana in the nadis and chakras and
help it to circulate smoothly. A balance of prana that flows
unimpeded in the body will directly improve your physical and emotional health. It is possible to focus on specific chakras during yoga practice to enhance their energy.

Yoga practice encourages kundalini energy (see page
23) to awaken and rise up the central nadi (sushumna). As
the energy reaches each chakra, the yogi experiences a specific spiritual state. This process may take many years or
lifetimes, with kundalini rising and falling before it finally
reaches its goal.

Yoga teachings advise that, as energy rises to the level
of each chakra, the yogi may acquire special powers known
as siddhis. The siddhi associated with ajna chakra, for example,
is telepathy. Rather than exploiting these siddhis the yogi
must use them with moderation and restraint in order to
attain enlightenment.

## Chakra meditation

Visualizing the chakras can be an effective aid to meditation (see Chapter 7) and a great way to try to "tune into"
their energy to bring particular benefits. Meditating upon
muladhara (at the perineum), for example, brings release
from physical and emotional tension as well as good
health. When meditating upon a certain chakra, try to visualize its colour at the appropriate place on your body
(imagine a wheel spinning brightly). Each time you
inhale, imagine drawing energy into the chakra. On each
exhalation let the energy radiate outward from the chakra.

If you feel inspired to use mantras during meditation,
each chakra has its own "seed" (bija) mantra that can be
chanted or repeated silently (sahasrara and ajna share the
seed mantra OM). The Sanskrit letters that appear on the
petals of the symbolic lotus flowers can also be used as
mantras. These and all the other specific characteristics of
each chakra are given on the chart on the following pages.

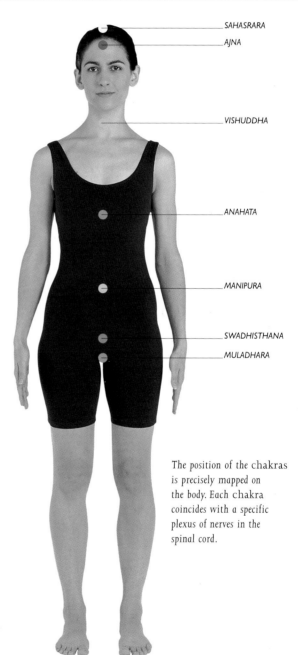

SAHASRARA
AJNA
VISHUDDHA
ANAHATA
MANIPURA
SWADHISTHANA
MULADHARA

*The position of the chakras
is precisely mapped on
the body. Each chakra
coincides with a specific
plexus of nerves in the
spinal cord.*

| | | | |
|---|---|---|---|
| CHAKRA NAME AND CHARACTERISTICS | *Sahasrara* (known as *nirvana chakra* in the Buddhist tradition) is represented by the full-blossomed lotus, which faces skyward and represents self-realization. Strictly speaking, *sahasrara* is not a *chakra,* but the point at which the physical body is transcended. | *Ajna* is also known as the third eye or the guru *chakra* (the latter name is derived from the fact that a student may receive telepathic communication from his guru via this *chakra*) and is associated with *manas* (mind), the face, eyes, nose, sinus and pituitary gland. | *Vishuddha* means "purity" and is where the nectar of immortality is produced. *Vishuddha* points forward and is associated with the lungs, neck, throat, vocal chords and jaw, as well as with knowledge, discrimination, humility and expression. |
| EXTERNAL LOCATION | Crown of the head | Forehead – between the eyes | Throat |
| INTERNAL LOCATION | Pineal gland | Pituitary gland | Thyroid gland |
| NUMBER AND COLOUR OF PETALS | One thousand white or golden petals | Two deep blue, pale grey or white petals | Sixteen sky-blue petals |
| MANTRA ON PETALS | Entire Sanskrit alphabet | *Ham* and *ksham* | Sixteen vowels of Sanskrit |
| SEED MANTRA | OM | OM | *Ham* |
| ELEMENT | Nothingness | Supreme element | Ether |
| MANIFEST APPEARANCE | Light and shapeless | Colourless oval | Smoky violet and round |
| SENSE | Higher mind | Intuition | Hearing |
| WORKING ORGAN | The five bodies (*koshas*) of man: one physical, the others subtle | Brain | Mouth |
| ANIMAL | None | None | White elephant – symbol of stren |
| DEITIES | Shiva, Para-Brahma | Parama-Shiva and Hakini | Ardhanarishvara and Shakini |
| *SIDDHI* (SPECIAL POWER) | Unity with the Absolute | Telepathy | Expression of being and oneness |
| LEVEL OF AWARENESS | Beyond awareness – pure being | Sixth plane of awareness – self-realization, knowledge of being | Fifth plane of awareness – expression of being |
| MEDITATE ON *CHAKRA* FOR: | Liberation of the mind; pure being | Unity and psychic guidance | Knowledge of the past |

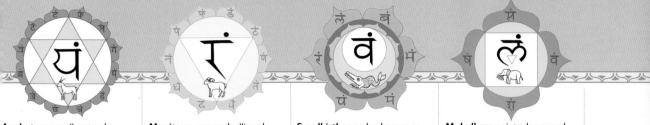

| **Anahata** means "unstruck sound" – the vibration of the universe (OM) is heard here. The body parts associated with this *chakra* are the heart, lungs, ribcage and upper back. This *chakra* points forward and is associated with ambition, hope, love, compassion and devotion. | **Manipura** means the "jewel city". The *chakra* points forward and is associated with the abdomen, back, stomach, spleen and digestive system, as well as immortality, fame, will-power and control. It is responsible for what we call "gut reactions" in everyday life. | **Swadhisthana**, also known as spleen *chakra*, points forward and is associated with the hands, reproductive organs, kidneys and bladder. It is the centre for creativity, sexual energy and emotion and is associated with reproduction, and all body fluids, including blood and saliva. | **Muladhara** points downward connecting to earth and is linked with the legs and the dense parts of the body, such as the bones and the teeth. Anxieties about basic physical survival, including food, shelter, safety and money, may be stored in this area. |
|---|---|---|---|
| Centre of chest | Navel | Over the spleen | Perineum, between the anus and genitals |
| Thymus | Near the adrenal glands (solar plexus) | Lumbosacral junction | Coccygeal-spinal junction |
| Twelve green or blue petals | Ten yellow petals | Six orange petals | Four red petals |
| Ka to ttha | *Dam, dham, nam, tam, tham, dam, dham, nam, pam, pham* | *Bam, bham, mam, yam, ram, lam* | *Vam, sham, kham, sam* |
| *Yam* | *Ram* | *Vam* | *Lam* |
| Air | Fire | Water | Earth |
| Smoky/invisible six-pointed star | Vermillion triangle | White crescent moon | Yellow square |
| Touch | Sight | Taste | Smell |
| Hands | Feet | Genitals | Anus |
| Antelope – symbol of speed | Ram – symbol of fiery energy | Crocodile – symbol of fertility | Elephant – symbol of strength |
| Isha and Kakini | Rudra and Lakini | Vishnu and Rakini | Brahma and Dakini |
| Unity of consciousness | Inspired teaching | Power of speech | Power of speech |
| Fourth plane of awareness – moving beyond the self | Third plane of awareness – formation of being | Second plane of awareness – reproduction of being | First plane of awareness – physical being |
| Spiritual and divine attainment | Transcending physical desires | Detachment from sensual pleasures and ego | Health and release of tension in physical body and mind |

# yoga now

Although yoga has its origins in ancient India, its methods and purposes are universal, relying not on cultural background, faith or deity, but simply on the individual. Yoga has become important in the lives of many contemporary Westerners, sometimes as a way of improving the health and fitness of the body, but also as a means of personal and spiritual development.

## Why do we need yoga?

Human nature has not changed all that much since the origins of yoga. We still ask the same questions about the meaning of life that people did thousands of years ago. In both the East and the West, the answers to such questions have been supplied over the ages by religion, philosophy, superstition and science. However, in the 21st-century industrialized West, religious beliefs have dwindled and many people feel dissatisfied with science – as a result we often feel spiritually "lost". Yoga offers a secular practice that can also meet our spiritual needs. As Swami Satyananda Saraswati says, "Yoga is not an ancient myth buried in oblivion. It is the most valuable inheritance of the present. It is the essential need of today and the culture of tomorrow."

### YOGA FOR CHILDREN

In India, some children begin yoga from the age of five. The benefits of improved health, fitness and concentration are well-documented, and now many forward-thinking schools in the West are beginning to teach yoga to children. This practice has been shown to enhance self-confidence, self-reliance, academic performance and the ability to cope with stressful situations, such as exams. The ethical disciplines of *yama* and *niyama* (see page 19) can also provide a moral framework for a child's life, regardless of cultural or religious background.

Hatha yoga is ideally suited to modern Westerners. Its structure is such that it starts with the very basics of how we experience existence – the physical body – and works inward. Increasingly, we fail to use our bodies enough or we have lifestyles that abuse them. Most of us suffer from back or joint pain at some stage, and many aspects of modern life – for example, sitting down for long periods of time to drive, watch television or work at a computer – place strains upon the body for which it is ill-prepared. We use medication to mask pain without bothering to establish its underlying cause. The flexibility and sensitivity that we had as children is lost as we gradually shut down our innate awareness of our bodies.

The strengthening, purifying and energizing practices of yoga can lead you back to a more complete awareness of yourself. It does not matter what kind of shape your body is in when you start your practice: just having a body – being alive – is a sufficient qualification for doing yoga. Then, having cultivated physical awareness, Hatha yoga aims to move on to develop higher levels of awareness. This physical route to spirituality is Hatha yoga's most unique and effective feature, and one which also marks the difference between yoga exercises and, say, gymnastics or Pilates.

## The benefits of yoga

Yoga practice is associated with physical, emotional and, ultimately, spiritual benefits. You may notice some benefits, such as increased flexibility and calm, early on in your yoga practice, while others may appear more slowly as you cultivate a new awareness of your body and mind.

The physical benefits of yoga include increased strength, suppleness and stamina. Unlike many sports and fitness routines, yoga works on all the body's muscles – this avoids overtraining specific muscle groups, a practice which can lead to injuries. Yoga enhances your balance, posture, agility and grace. It also cleanses and conditions internal systems and enhances bodily processes, such as digestion.

An emphasis on breathing techniques helps you to breathe better – deeper and more fully – even when you are not practising yoga. This leads to clarity and stillness of mind which, in turn, leads to improved concentration. You may also find that yoga helps to reduce anxiety, emotional tension and mood swings.

Yoga can help to alleviate or eliminate specific physical symptoms or ailments, such as PMS, headache, backache, stress, insomnia, asthma and irritable bowel syndrome. Under the guidance of a specialist teacher, yoga can aid the management of or recovery from more serious conditions, such as cancer, HIV, arthritis, multiple sclerosis and other degenerative diseases.

Most importantly, yoga is a personal path of discovery for each of us. Its particular and unique relevance to you will become apparent as you begin your practice.

*Yoga is a discipline that has relevance to everyone, regardless of age experience or background. These children from the Indian state of Assam are practising yoga as part of their school day.*

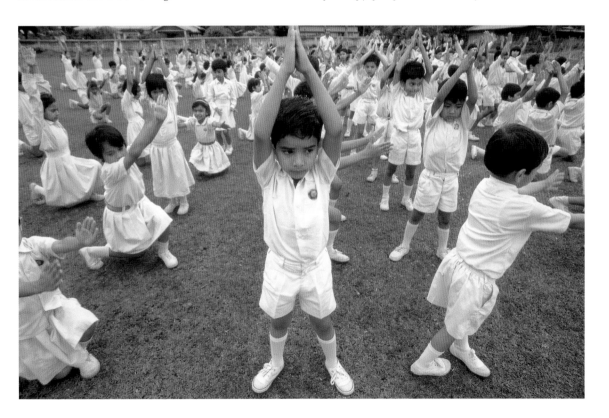

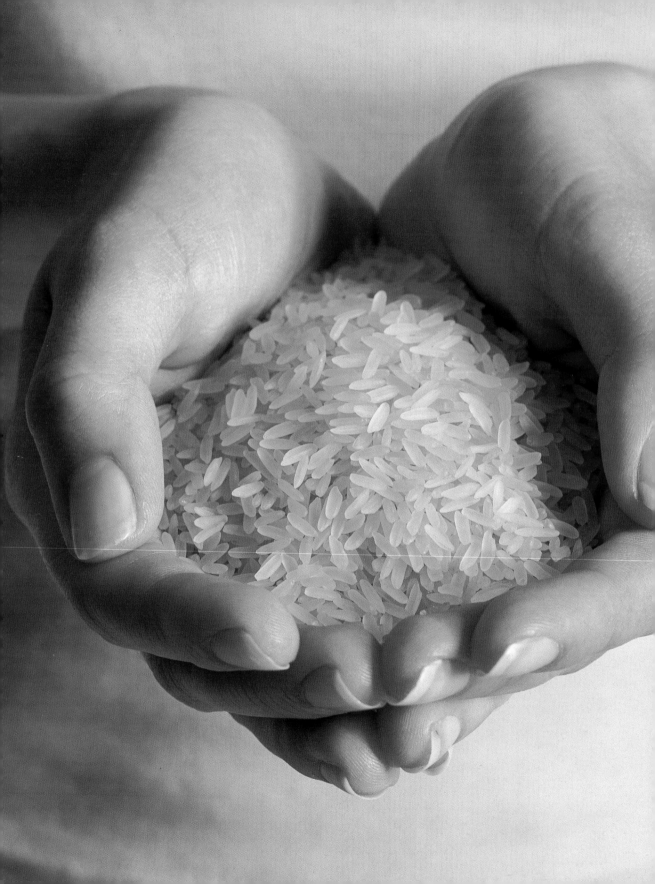

# the yoga diet

In the modern Western world we are fortunate to have access to an abundance of food – far more than we actually need. Nevertheless, our diet is frequently impoverished. Many of the foods that we eat are high in saturated fat, sugar, salt and flavourings, and lacking in fibre, vitamins, minerals and trace elements. Part of the reason for this is that modern food production involves extensive processing and refining techniques, which strip food of its natural goodness and introduce artificial ingredients that are designed to enhance flavour and shelf-life.

This chapter explains the dietary guidelines of yoga and their relation to Ayurveda – traditional Indian medicine. The diet advocates eating a variety of wholesome and nutritious foods that are tailored to your individual needs. By adopting this diet you can make significant improvements to your health and well-being.

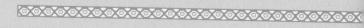

# the influence of the three gunas

The yogic approach to diet shares its origins with Ayurveda – the traditional Indian system of medicine. Both teach that the cosmos originates in the interactions of the three primal qualities known as *gunas*. These three qualities are *rajas* (energy), *tamas* (stasis) and *sattva* (harmony and balance). The *gunas* are present in everything: the air, the earth, animals, plants, people, food – even inanimate objects.

Each of the three *gunas* has a its own character. *Rajas* is hot, fiery, energetic and forceful. *Tamas* is slow, cool, inert and sustained. *Sattva* is pure, wholesome and clear; it is lucidity, a balance of *tamas* and *rajas*. Although all three *gunas* are present in each of us, one always predominates and influences all of our actions, thoughts and desires. It is not until we reach enlightenment (see pages 14–15), that we finally transcend the influence of the *gunas* and become free.

The yogic diet aims to balance the *gunas* through the foods we eat. In any food all three *gunas* are present, with one predominating. The balance of *gunas* can also alter in food; for example, a fresh pear is *sattvic*, but if cooked or allowed to over-ripen, its *tamasic* quality increases.

## Finding a balance

Strictly speaking, the basis of a yoga diet should be wholesome, nutritious *sattvic* foods. However, this is prescribed by the texts for those living a life devoted entirely to yoga. For the rest of us, we should identify which *guna* is dominant in our own particular case. This is determined by a range of factors, including our job, our personality and even the climate in which we live.

The process of identifying your dominant *guna* is complex and, for a detailed understanding, you will need to consult an Ayurvedic practitioner. But on a basic level you can try to adjust your dietary habits in relation to your personality and environment. If you are *rajasic* in character – fiery and energetic – you may need to eat *sattvic* and *tamasic* foods to achieve *sattva* (balance). If you

are feeling hot, stressed or overworked, you should also decrease the amount of *rajasic* foods in your diet. If you live in a cold climate and you have a sedentary job, you may need to eat more heating *rajasic* foods.

You can work toward achieving *sattva* – balance. Dietary changes should be made in conjunction with *asana* practice (which also helps you to achieve *sattva*).

## Sattvic food

*Sattvic* foods encourage balance in body and mind. By eating plenty of *sattvic* foods we can enjoy a peaceful mind within a fit body, and a harmonious flow of energy

### TAILORING YOUR DIET

Unlike Western principles of diet, which advocate similar dietary habits for everyone, a yogic diet must be tailored to individual character, physique and circumstances. Even if you find it difficult to identify your dominant *guna*, try experimenting with different foods to see what effect they have on the way you feel. Which foods make you feel clear-headed and energetic? Which foods make you feel stressed, excitable or jittery? And which ones make you feel slow and sluggish?

Regular *asana* practice often leads people into a greater sensitivity to the needs of their body and the effects that various foods have upon them.

between the two. *Sattvic* foods include grains, cereals, wholemeal bread, fresh fruit, fruit juice, fresh vegetables, milk, butter, cheese, honey, nuts, seeds, herbs (including herbal teas) and water.

## Tamasic food

*Tamasic* foods tend to be acidic, dry or old. In full-time yoga practice *tamasic* foods are to be avoided because of the spiritual harm that they cause. However, Ayurveda recognizes that eating *tamasic* foods may have a calming effect on an individual who is predominantly *rajasic*. *Tamasic* foods include mushrooms, meat, onion, garlic, fermented food, such as vinegar, reheated food and over-ripe or stale foods. Alcohol is also *tamasic*. *Sattvic* food that is fried in oil becomes more *tamasic*.

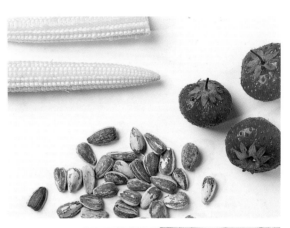

## Rajasic food

*Rajasic* foods tend to be hot, bitter or sour, or dry or salty. If you have a *rajasic* temperament, eating these foods can make you feel more restless or stressed. On the other hand, if you are feeling sluggish and lethargic they can give you increased energy. *Rajasic* foods include coffee, chocolate, tea, salt, fish, eggs, chilli peppers, and strong herbs and spices.

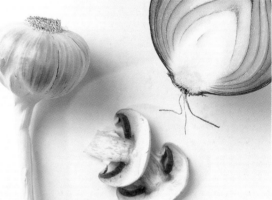

## The benefits of balancing the *gunas*

Eating a balanced yogic diet that takes account of the influence of the three *gunas* helps to keep your body slender and improve flexibility and physical well-being. A yogic diet increases the positive influence of *prana* (see pages 20–23) in your body, and makes your mind clear and focused. The yoga diet contains all the necessary elements to sustain, heal and develop the body without burdening it with excess waste or toxins.

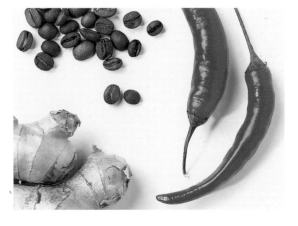

*Foods that are primarily sattvic in nature include fresh fruit and vegetables, and seeds (top); tamasic foods include garlic, onions and mushrooms (middle); and foods that are rajasic include coffee, ginger and chillies (bottom).*

# diet in practice

Yoga practitioners have followed the same dietary principles for thousands of years. They advocate a balance of pure and nutritious foods that should be eaten in moderation. According to the *Hathayoga Pradipika* (see pages 16–17), we should not eat so much that we are completely full, but instead should leave the stomach one quarter empty after a meal. We should also be in a calm and relaxed frame of mind when we eat.

The yogic term for the physical body (as opposed to the subtle body; see page 21) is *anamaya kosha*, which literally means "the food sheath". According to the *Chandogya Upanishad* (see page 17), the coarsest part of the food that we eat is eliminated from the body by the digestive system, the less coarse part is turned into flesh and the subtle part becomes the mind. This is why it is so important to pay attention to what you eat – you are what you eat. Food is not only fuel to keep you going through the day, it becomes part of your very being.

An important aspect of the yogic diet is moderation in eating. As the *Bhagavad Gita* (see page 17) says, "Yoga is not for him who over-eats, nor for he who fasts excessively." In the developed world where extreme diets, food fads and eating disorders are common, it is important to take note of these simple teachings. Furthermore, many of us eat while we are working or watching television rather than giving our attention to the food in front of us. We should take the time to eat slowly and chew food properly to aid digestion.

The yoga diet does not simply prescribe a specific range of foods to be eaten or avoided. Instead it sets out a range of underlying general principles, such as the three *gunas* (see pages 32–3) and vegetarianism, which can be adapted to our individual circumstances.

## GENERAL GUIDELINES

- Eat foods that are in a natural state, such as raw fruit and vegetables. Ideally, the food you eat should be freshly harvested. Supermarkets often import produce from other parts of the world, which necessitates it being refrigerated for long periods.
- Avoid foods that have been treated in ways that preserve them (for example, irradiated foods) and choose organically-grown produce instead. An increase in organic farming methods makes it easier than ever before to buy naturally-produced foods.
- Avoid processed food, white flour, sugar and convenience or "fast" foods (pre-cooked meals or food in tins, jars and bottles).
- Avoid foods that contain colouring, added sugar or salt, and modified starch or fats. Check food labels before you buy (laws on labelling are increasingly stringent).
- Eat as many fresh fruit and vegetables as possible. Cooking vegetables destroys vitamin and enzyme content, so you should try to eat some raw vegetables every day.

## Vegetarianism

The yogic diet is a lacto-vegetarian one, which means that it is made up entirely of non-animal foods with the exceptions of milk, cheese, yogurt, butter, eggs and honey. Some branches of yoga advocate a vegan diet in which no milk or milk products, eggs, honey or any other animal products should be eaten. Other branches of yoga, such as Tantric yoga, allow practitioners to eat meat, but this is unusual. The rationale behind a vegetarian diet is *ahimsa* – the yogic principle of non-harm and non-violence to all living things.

Apart from the ethical approach of *ahimsa* there are other reasons for following a vegetarian diet. Evidence suggests that a predominantly vegetarian diet is good for our health. Meat protein takes a long time to digest and tends to be difficult for the kidneys and liver to eliminate. Meat also contains a high proportion of uric acid, which has been linked to problems such as stiffness and joint pain. In addition, animals may be fed with hormones and antibiotics that can enter our bodies when we eat meat.

Contrary to popular belief, most vegetarian diets supply adequate amounts of protein for the body's needs – pulses, nuts and seeds are all rich in protein – and anyway many Westerners (vegetarians included) eat far more protein than we actually need.

Many people ask whether it is essential to be a vegetarian in order to practice yoga. Although the practice of *ahimsa* is an ideal one, yoga does not demand overnight conversions or changes in lifestyle. Indeed, Patanjali's eight-fold path (see page 19) fully acknowledges the difficulties we come across in living according to yogic principles. And if you are not a vegetarian, you will still gain benefits from other aspects of your yoga practice. A gradual approach – eating more vegetarian meals week-by-week or month-by-month – will allow your body time to adjust. You may find vegetarian foods a pleasant source of culinary inspiration – a valuable introduction to a broader diet.

Some people find that, having incorporated *asana* and *pranayama* (breath control) into their lives, they want to broaden their yoga practice to include the principles of social and personal conduct (*yamas* and *niyamas*; see page 19) – this naturally leads them to stop wanting to eat meat.

*Asana* practice in particular can encourage a heightened awareness of the effect of meat and substances such as caffeine and alcohol on the mind and body. (You may also find that *asana* practice sharpens your sense of taste and smell, and reduces your cravings for sugary, spicy and salty foods.)

*The yogic diet favours food that is grown in harmony with the natural environment. This is in line with the principle of ahimsa (non-harm; see page 19).*

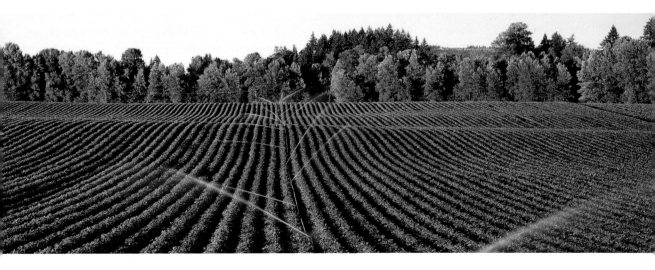

# water – the source of life

Water is vital to the healthy functioning of the human body. Without water – which accounts for around eighty per cent of our body mass – the body cannot effectively eliminate toxins and waste matter or grow new tissue. Drinking the right amount of water is particularly important as you begin *asana* practice. The body responds to *asana* by eliminating built-up waste deposits, and it needs plenty of water to flush out the system.

Most of us simply do not drink enough pure water – it is possible to live in a state of permanent semi-dehydration without even realizing it. Dehydration can cause headaches, bad breath and many other minor health problems. Drinking tea and coffee throughout the day – as many people do – is a poor way of maintaining fluid intake. Tea and coffee are both *rajasic* (see pages 32–3) and do not have the same rehydrating effects as plain water. They have a diuretic effect on the body, which means that they increase the output of urine and the overall loss of water from the body. They also contain caffeine, which is a stimulant and places stress on the body.

### Signs of dehydration

If you regularly notice any of the following signs, you should increase the amount of water that you drink on a daily basis: your saliva is sticky; you feel weak, lethargic or fatigued; you don't urinate very often and when you do, your urine is dark yellow or orange. (You should consult your doctor if you suffer from severe fatigue or urinary problems.)

Another sign of dehydration is dry skin – modern centrally-heated and air-conditioned homes often dry out the skin. Rather than trying to rehydrate the skin from the outside by applying moisturizing creams, rehydrate it from the inside by drinking more water.

### Maintaining your fluid intake

To keep your body properly hydrated you need to drink approximately 2 litres (about 4 pints) of water a day – more if you are sweating a lot (owing to exercise, fever or living in a hot climate) or have recently suffered from diarrhoea or vomiting.

To get into the habit of drinking more water you can drink a glass every hour from the time you wake up to the time you go to sleep. Another way is to drink as much water as you comfortably can (about a litre, if possible) first thing in the morning, and then smaller amounts throughout the day. Ideally, you should drink pure, uncarbonated water on an empty stomach because this maximizes the water's cleansing and hydrating potential. The body treats other drinks, including any type of "flavoured" water, as something it needs to digest differently in order to extract nutritional benefit.

You can increase your overall intake of fluids by drinking herb teas, fruit and vegetable juices, and milk and vegetable milks (coconut, soya, rice milk and so on) and by eating water-rich foods, such as fruit and vegetables. However, there is no substitute for drinking plenty of plain, pure water. Carbonated water is made bubbly by the addition of carbon dioxide (the same gas that you exhale as waste on every out-breath). Although the addition of gas might make water seem more appetizing, it can also cause discomfort and wind. It is inadvisable to drink lots of water with meals as this can dilute the digestive fluids and impede nutrient absorption.

Never try to lose weight by cutting down on the amount of water you drink – this is extremely damaging to the body. In fact, drinking plenty of water can sometimes help to overcome weight problems and, strangely enough, fluid retention. This is because we often retain water owing to a toxic or mineral imbalance in the body. By increasing the amount of water you drink, you can resolve this imbalance.

## The quality of water

All drinking water contains a combination of different minerals which affects its chemical constitution and flavour. Most bottled waters are slightly alkaline (more than pH7) – such waters are usually referred to as "hard". Most people consider hard water to be more palatable than soft water (some of the softer mineral waters are said to taste slightly soapy). Tap water, which varies in alkalinity depending on where you live, is always chemically treated and may also have fluoride added. Although drinking tap water is better than nothing, it is advisable to drink the best quality bottled water that you can afford.

A side-effect of *asana* practice is a refinement of your senses of taste and smell. This means that you may detect variations in the taste of different types of water – just as you can with wine. Try buying a range of bottled waters and tasting them side by side – you will find that they each have their own unique character. You may begin to appreciate the taste of certain brands of mineral water and become quite a connoisseur!

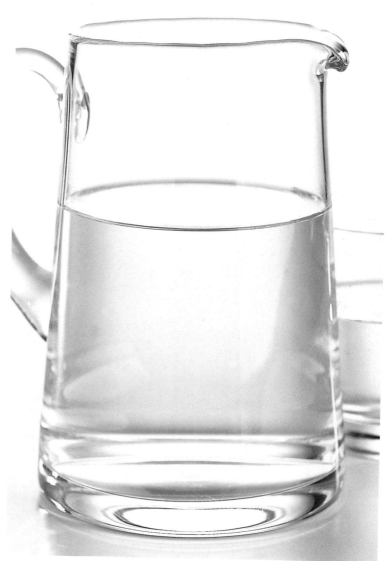

*Water is the simplest substance that we can ingest and yet one of the most fundamental to our well-being – our digestion and metabolism depend upon it. After asana practice, wait 15 minutes or so before drinking water, as this is when it will be most beneficial in cleansing your system.*

# fasting for health

Fasting is an extremely effective way to cleanse and purify the body and mind. A fast allows the entire digestive system time to rest, and the energy that you would normally use to digest and absorb food is instead used to repair and strengthen all of your body systems. In addition, many people find that fasting makes them feel particularly alert and clear-headed, enabling them to focus better and achieve longer periods of concentration or meditation.

Fasting is an act of self-discipline that should be carefully managed. Although austerity and self-control are important ideals, yoga does not condone extreme self-deprivation. A fast should be used only to cleanse your system and restore balance to your body. Fasting should be avoided by anyone who is unwell, pregnant, breastfeeding or taking prescribed medication, unless under strict supervision. Fasts should not be held too frequently (many people find that fasting seasonally is sufficient).

Fasting should not be considered a quick way to lose weight. A weight-loss diet involves a long-term plan of calorie restriction and dietary modification. During a fast, your food intake is restricted for a few days only, and this does not make the body shed fat.

### Going on a fast

A short fast can last between one and three days. A one-day fast can rest the digestive system, but a longer fast is needed for the body to undergo proper detoxification. If you want to fast for more than a day, seek the advice of a herbalist or naturopath. As fasting involves some disruption to your everyday life, plan to fast during a period when you don't have to work and are able to devote your time to rest.

Two days before a fast, you should prepare your body by simplifying your diet to a few basic

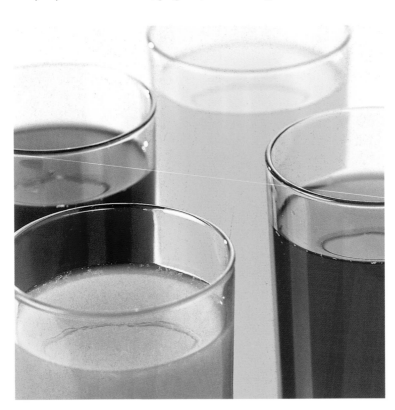

*Freshly-prepared juice, which is rich in vitamins and minerals, is easily digested and absorbed and doesn't place any stress on the body. It is an excellent drink while fasting.*

ingredients. Instead of your normal meals, eat a light diet of fruit, vegetables and perhaps some yogurt. Then on the day of your fast, eliminate all solid foods and drink either fruit or vegetable juice (don't mix them – our body uses different enzymes to digest them). Drink up to about 4 litres (about 7–8 pints) of juice a day and try to "chew" it rather than simply gulp it down – this aids digestion. It is possible to fast exclusively on water but if you would like to do this, you should seek supervision from a herbalist or naturopath, at least for your first time.

You will find that you don't have very much energy during a fast and, for this reason, you should avoid strenuous exercise. A gentle practice of yoga postures, however, can help to speed up the process of detoxification. Walking is another good form of gentle exercise and can also act as a natural aid to meditation (fasting is an excellent time to devote to concentration and meditation as the mind may feel sharper and more acute than usual).

During a fast, toxins and impurities are released from the body through all the organs of elimination, including the skin. You should wash regularly to keep the skin fresh and clean. Try brushing the skin with a natural vegetable bristle brush, which helps to remove dead skin cells and stimulate the circulation and the nervous system. Avoid using any type of skin product during your fast, in particular antiperspirant, which blocks up the skin's pores. You may experience skin eruptions as the body goes through its internal cleaning process, but these should clear up in a couple of days.

## Side-effects of fasting

It is completely normal to feel a little cold or shivery while fasting, so make sure that you dress yourself warmly. However, you may have any of the following side-effects: headaches, bad breath, a coated tongue, dizziness, mild palpitations and nausea.

Most of these side-effects are minor, but if you suffer from strong palpitations or breathing problems, then you

### PREPARING JUICES

Juices have the best nutritional and *pranic* (see pages 20–23) qualities when freshly pressed, and can be an important part of your diet when fasting. You can buy unsweetened, organic juices from supermarkets and health-food shops, but the best option is to make them freshly at home.

Make sure that the fruit or vegetables you choose are firm, fresh and thoroughly washed. If possible, buy organic produce or harvest your own. Discard produce that is bruised, blemished, over- or under-ripe (although over-ripe fruit yields more juice, it is less nutritious). The addition of a small amount of lemon juice to a freshly-made juice will stop it turning brown when it comes into contact with the air.

Left-over juice can be stored in a sealed container in the fridge but, as juice doesn't keep long, it is best to make it frequently in small amounts and drink it all at once. Juices are best drunk at room temperature, rather than cold.

should seek the advice of a doctor, herbalist or naturopath immediately and come off the fast slowly.

## Breaking a fast

Breaking your fast should be a slow and gentle process so that your body has a chance to re-adjust. On the last evening of a fast, eat one type of fresh fruit, such as grapes (avoid acidic fruits such as oranges). Then, the following morning, at around 10am, eat some more fruit and perhaps a small bowl of yogurt. Have a similar meal in the evening at around 5pm. The next day your diet should consist of raw vegetables and salads. The following day you can add rice, or another grain, and some steamed vegetables. After this you can return to eating normally.

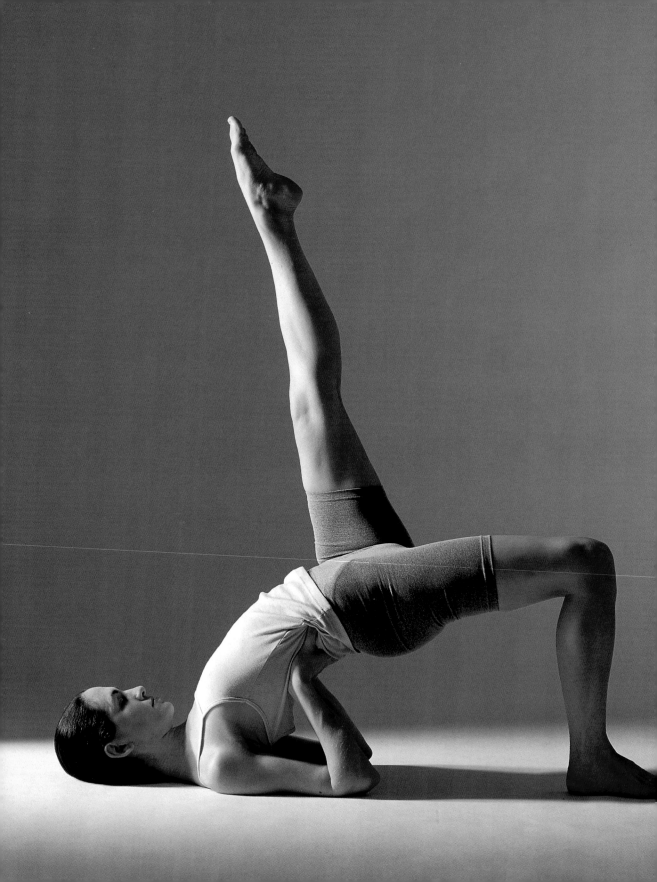

# understanding posture

The best introduction that you can have to yoga postures is through classes that are taught by an experienced teacher. Owing to the explosion in popularity of yoga in the West there is a now a great diversity of classes to choose from. This chapter describes the differences between some of the principal styles of yoga and how to go about choosing the right class for you.

Having experienced yoga in a class, your next step should be to start developing your own posture practice at home. Self-practice offers you the opportunity to integrate what you have learned in a class with your personal understanding of your body. In this way you move from following the instructions of a teacher to beginning your own inner journey. This chapter suggests ways of starting and maintaining self-practice, as well as other useful skills that will help you to begin a lifelong practice of yoga.

# starting *asana* practice

*Asana*, meaning posture, is the mainstay of Hatha yoga (see page 15). For most Westerners, posture practice is the first experience they have of yoga and for many it provides a starting point for meditation and spiritual discovery. Through *asana* practice you will develop a greater sensitivity to and awareness of your physical self. The subtle connections between the mind and the body are awakened, and you will learn how to control and regulate your breathing, both when you are moving and when you are still.

The practice of *asana* can be hugely beneficial for everyone, no matter what your age, background, beliefs, lifestyle, or physical and mental state. However, the way in which you practise *asana* should be determined by a variety of factors such as how strong you are, how much time you have available and also what you hope to achieve from yoga (see page 46). Bear in mind that yoga is a system of personal development and, for it to be effective, you should adapt your *asana* practice to your own unique needs and lifestyle. For example, the *asana* practice of an athletic 21-year-old might be very different from that of a 37-year-old working mother with back problems. Try to be aware of your physical limitations and work within them. You should feel comfortable and confident in a posture before you attempt a more difficult variation; take careful note of the precautions given with the *asanas* in Chapter 4. Yoga is a gentle process – it is not about forcing yourself through pain barriers.

### Getting started

If you are just beginning yoga, it can be really beneficial to attend classes to learn some of the basic postures. Learning from a teacher is easier than trying to learn on your own – at least at first. However, even while you are attending classes, try to practise on your own at home using chapters 4, 5 and 8 of this book to prompt your memory of the postures and extend your repertoire. If you have a severe or chronic medical condition, an injury, or if you are pregnant, you must find a good teacher who can guide you toward a practice that meets your needs.

You need very few props for your *asana* practice. A specially designed yoga mat may help you to grip the floor in some of the standing postures, such as down-facing dog (see page 62), and if you are stiff in the lower back or hamstrings, a specially-designed hard foam block or a large book (a telephone directory, for example), can help support you in postures such as the sitting forward bend (see page 72). A folded, single, firmly-woven blanket can be helpful for postures such as the shoulderstand (see pages 86–7). Wear soft comfortable clothes that allow complete freedom of movement, and go barefoot.

### Charting your progress

An excellent way to monitor your *asana* practice is to keep a yoga diary. Make a note of the date, the time you began your practice and the time you finished, as well as which postures you did and how long you stayed in each one. Make notes about how the postures felt: did they cause you any discomfort, did you find them easy or difficult and did you enjoy them? It can be very encouraging to look back over weeks or months to see how your practice develops.

## GUIDELINES FOR POSTURE PRACTICE

- Make sure that you avoid eating before practising any *asanas* – leave an hour after a light snack and at least three hours after a heavy meal. You should avoid drinking anything, including water, during posture practice.

- Whether you learn yoga from a teacher or a book, follow the instructions for getting into a posture carefully. Do not fling or force yourself into a posture. Nothing in yoga should be violent, uncontrolled or careless. Don't expect to look exactly like the pictures in this book right away; just take care to follow the instructions.

- Breathe evenly and steadily through your nose throughout posture practice. As a general rule, breathe in during upward or lifting movements and breathe out during downward or twisting and folding movements.

- If something hurts, stop.

- Try to be "present" in a posture. Focus on the reality of it moment by moment and notice how it changes as you move.

- Trust yourself to explore a posture like an inquisitive child. Observe yourself, your habits and preferences, and the way you breathe in the pose as you enter it, as you hold it and as you come out of it. Never stop experimenting.

- Don't concentrate on one part of the body to the detriment of another part. Your whole body should work in harmony during a posture.

- Generally lift, lengthen and extend the body. The illustrations shown here demonstrate the correct and incorrect way to perform three *asanas*. Note how the incorrect versions show the body in a collapsed, compressed or rigid position. The correct versions show an open, extended and supported position. Full details of these *asanas* are given in Chapter 4.

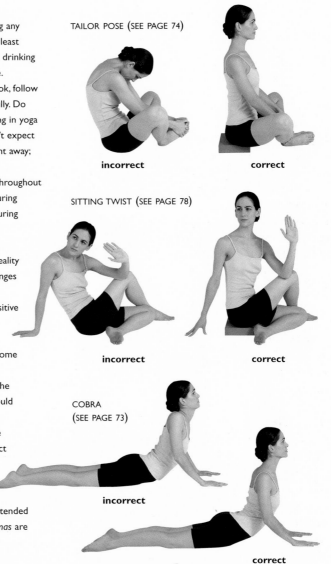

TAILOR POSE (SEE PAGE 74)

**incorrect**          **correct**

SITTING TWIST (SEE PAGE 78)

**incorrect**          **correct**

COBRA
(SEE PAGE 73)

**incorrect**

**correct**

# styles of yoga

The main type of yoga taught in the West is Hatha yoga (see page 15). Within the discipline of Hatha yoga there are several teaching styles that have been pioneered by individuals. All of them teach similar postures to those that appear in Chapter 4, but there are variations in the emphasis placed on different aspects of yoga. For example, some styles emphasize a dynamic performance of set sequences of postures; some concentrate on detailed work on alignment within individual postures; others include spiritual teaching or chanting. The descriptions below will help you to find a style of yoga that suits you.

### Iyengar yoga

B.K.S. Iyengar, who teaches all over the world, is renowned as one of the greatest living yogis (his institute is in Pune in western India). Iyengar yoga is popular in the West; its main characteristic is the precise physical alignment of each posture. Teachers of this style have extensive anatomical knowledge and are adept at dealing with injuries and physical problems. Various shaped blocks, bolsters, belts, blankets and other props are used to assist posture practice in Iyengar classes. Students learn *asana* first and then progress to breathing techniques. Overt spiritual teaching is unlikely in a beginners' class.

### Astanga vinyasa yoga

The word *astanga* means "eight-limbed" (after Patanjali's eight limbs of yoga; see page 19) and *vinyasa* means "linked". The *astanga vinyasa* style has been developed by Pattabhi Jois (born in 1915) at the *Astanga* Yoga Institute in Mysore, southern India. Students learn a series of postures in a particular order. The first series that students are taught is called the primary series; when this is mastered the second series and advanced series are taught. The postures within each series are connected by linking movements (*vinyasa*) to create a smooth, flowing sequence. A class that is advertised as "Mysore-style practice" means that students are expected to know the series of postures already and will be assisted by the teacher as appropriate.

Astanga vinyasa is a dynamic and physically demanding style of yoga and students are taught to use a strong breathing technique throughout their practice. Meditation is experienced through movement (ideal for people who find a traditional sitting meditation practice difficult or unappealing). *Astanga vinyasa* yoga is best suited to people who enjoy a physical challenge and are in good health. Classes often begin and end with group chanting of the *astanga* yoga mantras.

### Dynamic yoga

This is the name given to a strong flowing practice that is similar in style to *astanga vinyasa*. The main difference between dynamic yoga and *astanga vinyasa* is that the former is a modified version that does not teach postures in the primary, secondary and advanced series structure. The main teacher associated with dynamic yoga is the British yogi, Godfrey Deveraux.

### Jivamukti yoga

From the Sanskrit meaning "liberation while in the living body", *jivamukti* is a modern yoga method, developed from *astanga vinyasa* by David Life and Sharon Gannon and is currently taught at their yoga centre in New York. This is a strong dynamic style characterized by flowing sequences of postures (different from the series of postures that are used in *astanga vinyasa*), spiritual teaching and chanting, breathing and meditation. As with other dynamic forms, *jivamukti* yoga is physically demanding and generally suited to people who are injury-free and in a good state of health.

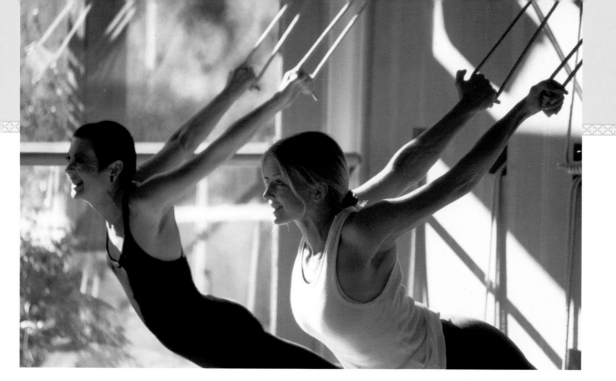

## Bikram's yoga

The pioneer of this style of yoga is Bikram Choudury, who was born in Calcutta in 1948 and who now practises in Beverly Hills, Los Angeles. Students are taught a sequence of 26 postures. A distinctive aspect of this style is that classrooms are heated to more than 100°F (38°C), recreating the Indian climate. Students sweat profusely, which is intended to speed up the cleansing effect of the postures and increase flexibility. You need to be reasonably fit for this style of yoga.

## Viniyoga

This style was developed by T.K.V. Desikachar in the 1960s from the teachings of his father Sri Krishnamacharya (the yogi who also taught B.K.S. Iyengar and Pattabhi Jois). Viniyoga is a gentle form of yoga which includes breathing and posture practice, as well as spiritual and philosophical teaching. It is usually taught one-to-one or in small groups. This amount of individual attention is ideal for people who are injured or recovering from illness.

## Sivananda yoga

Swami Sivananda developed this popular method of yoga and introduced it to the West in the 1950s. Sivananda

*Iyengar yoga is characterized by meticulous attention to detail within the postures. To assist correct body alignment, students in Iyengar classes use a variety of props including straps and ropes.*

yoga comprises 12 basic postures and variations or series based on these postures. Students learn breathing techniques and they may learn chanting. Spiritual teaching often plays an important role in Sivananda classes.

## Bihar yoga

The Bihar school of yoga in Munger, Bihar, India was founded by Swami Satyananda Saraswati in 1964. Swami Satyananda Saraswati was a student of Swami Sivananda and he travelled extensively in the West for many years. He and his disciples have written more than 80 books, many of which have become classic treatises on yoga.

Bihar yoga teachers have access to extensive training in all aspects of yoga. Classes have a similar feel to Sivananda yoga. General and beginners' classes are not likely to be physically demanding and may include spiritual or philosophical teaching. Some Bihar yoga teachers specialize in chanting or in the physiological effects of postures (the latter is known as yoga therapy). Bihar yoga teachers often run yoga classes for children.

# finding a yoga class

Students who are new to yoga can benefit greatly from attending classes where a teacher is on hand to provide instruction, support, encouragement and inspiration, and to demonstrate the subtler points of *asana* practice, such as using muscular locks (*bandhas*; see page 107) and breathing techniques. Perhaps the best piece of advice for choosing a yoga class is to experiment until you find one that suits your personal needs.

No one style of yoga is superior to another and it is as impossible – and undesirable – to teach a single correct method of yoga as it is to teach a single correct way to paint or to compose music. You may even find that some methods appear to contradict others on specific points or details – don't let this worry you, as every style of yoga leads to the same goal.

The first step in choosing the right yoga class is to work out what it is that you would like to experience in yoga. For example, are you looking for a spiritual discipline, or a way to tone your muscles, recover from an injury or become more flexible or relaxed? Or are you simply interested in trying a new form of therapeutic exercise and personal development? Talk to a prospective yoga teacher about your needs and preferences before you sign up for a course. Don't hesitate to ask questions about a teacher's background and favoured style of yoga. You could even try a range of different classes on a drop-in basis to find one that matches your interests. If appropriate, look out for classes that cater for specific needs, such as classes for the over-50s or for pregnant women.

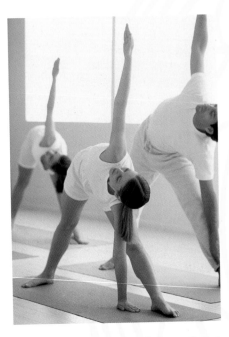

Try to find a yoga class that caters for between five and 15 people. In a small class a teacher can give students more individual help and attention.

Another factor to consider when choosing a class is how frequently it runs. Many students who are just beginning yoga find that attending one yoga class a week meets their needs, but as you become more experienced you may benefit from doing more classes (or combining practice in a class with self-practice). Advanced students, who already practice yoga daily at home, may benefit from attending yoga classes as and when they need to for encouragement, support and advice from a teacher.

## The venue

Yoga's increasing popularity makes it easy to find classes in a wide variety of venues – health clubs, gyms, community centres, church halls and, of course, purpose-built yoga centres. It is worth considering whether the yoga class is geared to the environment in which it is taught. For example, classes that are held in health clubs may concentrate on the physical side of yoga and neglect the spiritual aspects. Teaching yoga solely as a form of exercise has been criticised by some yoga practitioners. Although in some cases these criticisms may be justified,

## ATTENDING A YOGA CLASS

Yoga classes vary enormously, but here are some general guidelines on what to expect and how to prepare.

- At the beginning of the class the teacher will ask if anyone has an injury or a medical condition or if anyone is pregnant. You should inform your teacher of any health problems, even those that you consider trivial.
- Most classes last 90 minutes or more. Much of this time is spent doing posture practice (you may be taught some of the *asanas* in Chapter 4), but time is also spent on breathing practices and relaxation. The structure of posture practice varies greatly but may, for example, start with standing postures and progress to sitting and lying postures.

- Most classes will provide any necessary props such as mats and blocks, but you can also bring your own.
- You will need to practise in bare feet and wear soft, stretchy clothing that allows complete freedom of movement.
- As with any yoga practice, you should avoid eating before a class or drinking anything, including water, during a class.
- To derive the maximum benefits from a yoga class try to concentrate on your own practice rather than comparing yourself with fellow students. Try to be impartial rather than competitive or envious.
- Classes often end with a period of guided relaxation in which you lie in the corpse pose (see page 89) and focus on releasing tension from your body.

it is also true that many of us are increasingly disconnected or estranged from our bodies. If physical training provides a route back to physical – and eventually spiritual – awareness, then this is Hatha yoga at work.

Spiritual teaching may be more likely in classes set up by independent yoga teachers (rather than those in health clubs) or in specialist yoga centres. Decide which aspects of yoga are important to you and consider a venue with this in mind.

### The teacher

Choosing a teacher is a bit like choosing a friend: trust your judgment and you will know when it feels right. In practical terms, a good teacher allows for different levels of skill and understanding among students and creates a nurturing environment. Look for a teacher who gives clear instructions, corrects your postures on a one-to-one basis and responds readily to any queries or needs that you have. Teachers may correct postures verbally or by making physical adjustments to your body and by

demonstrating correct and incorrect versions of a posture to provide you with a visual guide.

There are several organizations that accredit yoga teachers (see page 139) and they may be able to supply a list of teachers working in your local area. However, although an accreditation certificate may provide a reassuring badge of competence, it is not necessarily a guarantee of a talented or sensitive teacher. Experiment by attending a variety of classes until you find the right teacher for you.

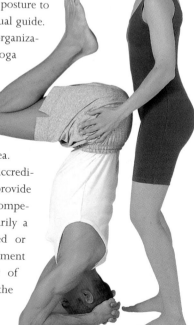

# self-practice

Many students attend yoga classes regularly for years but find it difficult or even impossible to take the next step – independent posture practice at home. Although you will learn a great deal from a teacher when starting out, you will experience most of yoga's benefits by practising alone. This is because, ultimately, yoga is a process of self-realization and you are the best expert on yourself. If you haven't started self-practice yet, you can use these guidelines as a way to begin.

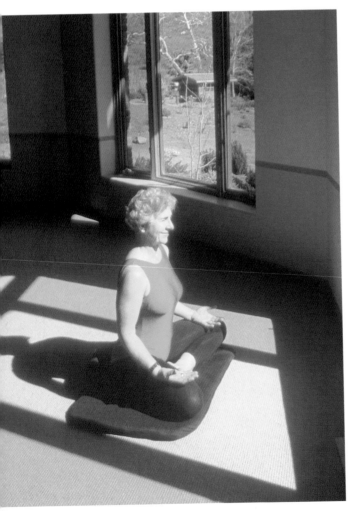

There are two main obstacles to self-practice. The first, and most obvious, is discipline (see box, opposite); the second, less obvious, but just as problematic, is lack of self-confidence. In virtually all aspects of our lives we are encouraged to rely upon experts. We consult them on everything from relationships and health to cookery and law. We often lose awareness of our instinct or intuition, with the result that, when we try to practise yoga in the absence of a teacher, we feel that our knowledge and experience is inadequate. Yet to benefit fully from yoga we must learn to be at one with and trust ourselves.

**Starting self-practice**

Try to cultivate the confidence to practise yoga on your own. You do not have to, nor should you, start off with a difficult pose, such as a headstand (see pages 84–5). Instead, you could begin with something quiet and straightforward, such as resting in child pose (see page 68), and simply observe how you feel.

You can start your self-practice by doing some of the postures in Chapter 4. This chapter does not provide an exhaustive list (there are said to be 840,000 yoga postures), but it does offer a reasonable range from which to choose. If you have been taking yoga classes, you will doubtless recognize many of the postures, although you may have been taught slightly different variations of some

*Self-practice is the key to long-lasting benefits in yoga. Start with postures that you feel confident about and use props such as blankets and mats to support you in a pose.*

of them. If you are new to yoga, do not feel daunted by the photographs – they are there to guide you. You should aim to make progress gradually.

Practising a variety of postures in sequence (see Chapter 5) gives a balanced structure to your practice. Choose sequences that suit your mood and energy levels: try something dynamic and energizing when you wake up in the morning and something relaxing after work. The gentle sequence on pages 96–7 is ideal for beginners.

Practise in a warm, quiet and clear space. A mirror leaned against the wall can be helpful to check occasionally that your body is correctly aligned. However, do avoid practising habitually in front of a mirror – this encourages you to focus on your external appearance instead of how you feel, which is much more important.

## How much and how often?

A total beginner will benefit from 15 minutes' practice, three to five days a week, increasing to 45-minute sessions after a few months. Eventually, you could aim to build up to an hour or more daily (this includes attending classes), with one rest day a week.

However, the wisdom of experience from practitioners and teachers suggests that not everyone responds well to rigid timetables. We are often urged to work to schedules in life but this can be counterproductive – if you feel that your self-practice has become an obligation, you may well be less motivated to do it.

Remember that yoga should be enjoyable and life-enhancing. Try to tailor your self-practice sessions to your needs. If your lifestyle is hectic, tiring or changeable, simply do what you can. For example, use meditation techniques instead of posture practice when you are physically exhausted. Take a long posture practice when you have plenty of time to yourself. A little yoga, practised often, is far better for you than no yoga at all, or even yoga practised when you would rather be doing something else.

### GETTING STARTED

Finding the discipline to start self-practice can be a major obstacle for many of us. Resolve to set a day for your first session and keep to it. Practice for a short period of, say, around 15 minutes. The most important thing is to establish the routine of doing yoga, so that it becomes part of your everyday life. Here are some techniques that may help you to start and maintain your practice. Different things work for different people – if one technique doesn't work, try another one instead.

• Give yourself a set time and place to practise.

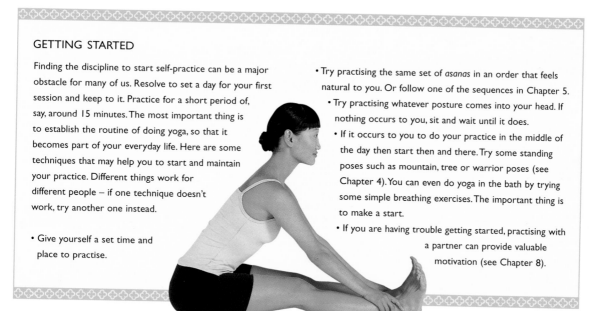

• Try practising the same set of *asanas* in an order that feels natural to you. Or follow one of the sequences in Chapter 5.

• Try practising whatever posture comes into your head. If nothing occurs to you, sit and wait until it does.

• If it occurs to you to do your practice in the middle of the day then start then and there. Try some standing poses such as mountain, tree or warrior poses (see Chapter 4). You can even do yoga in the bath by trying some simple breathing exercises. The important thing is to make a start.

• If you are having trouble getting started, practising with a partner can provide valuable motivation (see Chapter 8).

# overcoming problems

Starting self-practice isn't always easy, but once you have developed the confidence to make the transition from yoga in a class to yoga at home, you have passed a major milestone. Everybody will come across some difficulties in their yoga practice, but as you work through them, they form part of your learning experience. It can be helpful to be aware of some of the common problems that you might encounter during self-practice.

## Feelings of ambition

Once you have begun to master the postures in your self-practice, beware of excessive pride or ambition in performing them. It is the process of practising, rather than the attainment of a "perfect" pose, that is important. Trying to do very difficult postures without going through the preparatory stages is a form of impatient ambition, and by doing this you will cheat yourself of the full benefits of the posture. In yoga it is important to cultivate the ability to do things without undue attachment to the end results.

Years ago, I was in a class struggling with a posture, arching my back and twisting my rib cage to see if I could get my hands to meet around my back. The teacher said to me, "Don't rob Peter to pay Paul." Suddenly, I could see that in my ambition to get into the full posture, I was spoiling the rest of my good practice by holding my breath, letting my back collapse and generally straining to get those fingers to touch! There must be a balance between effort and ease. A yoga posture, according to the ancient texts, should be steady, firm and comfortable.

For many postures in Chapter 4, I have suggested easier modifications. You are not failing if you use these modifications. In fact, you will be practising intelligently by letting go of ambition.

## Self-criticism

You may also need to let go of self-criticism. Yoga does require detailed self-analysis, but this is very different from demoralizing self-criticism. It is common to feel that are you are not making progress fast enough, practising long enough or regularly enough, or simply that you are not very "good" at the postures. This is inverted ambition – by setting yourself unrealistic goals you make yourself feel defeated when you don't reach them. Remember – yoga is not about success or failure, but about personal development. Being able to stand on your head does not make you a yogi! Allow your observations of your self-practice to be accurate and impartial. If you find yourself being self-critical, bring your attention to your breathing to help still your mind.

## Powerful emotions

Our minds and our bodies are so intimately related that it is possible for emotions to be diverted from the mind and stored physically in the body. This is a useful coping mechanism in the short-term, but over a longer period of time it can become debilitating. Yoga helps to free stored emotions by opening the channels that connect the mind and spirit with the physical body. You may experience dramatic emotions during or after performing postures or breathing exercises. Don't be alarmed if you find yourself temporarily tearful, angry, frightened or even gloriously happy. This marks the letting go of emotions that may have been building up over a lifetime. Let yourself rest quietly in corpse pose (see page 89) or child pose (see page 68). Powerful emotions that are released during yoga practice will pass quite quickly, leaving you refreshed and unburdened. If you persistently experience these feelings, seek advice from a yoga therapist.

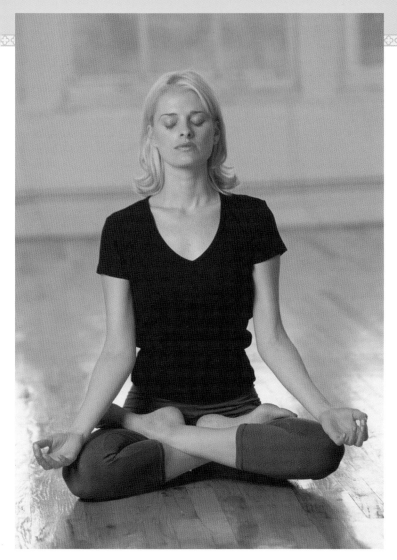

*Release yourself from egotistical thoughts during posture practice and concentrate on being in the moment. Be as non-judgmental about your practice as possible.*

Much more common, but less worrying, is muscular discomfort that occurs when you deepen into a posture. This should be embraced and moved with rather than resisted. Use your breath to develop a posture: ground yourself on your in-breath and release your body further on each out-breath. The working loose of muscular tension is ultimately a healing process.

If your practice causes you pain, do a gentler practice. When you notice you are resisting one posture, try another. Sometimes, understanding one posture can help you with another, even when they are apparently unrelated.

If you have an existing injury or illness, take care that your practice neither aggravates your condition nor ignores it. Go to a yoga teacher for help and advice, especially if you have acute or chronic pain.

**Pain and discomfort**

Generally speaking, it is not good to be in pain. Joint pain or any hard, sharp pain that makes you wince and pull away from a posture is usually a signal to stop. The cause may be emotional or physical – the two are closely related. If you experience pain, be extremely careful. Exit the pose slowly and consider what you were doing to produce the pain – modify your practice accordingly.

**Technique**

Finally, try to exist "in the moment" during your self-practice. Don't distract yourself by wishing your body was different or by remembering how it used to be or anticipating how it might be in the future. It is only by understanding your current experience that you can hope to progress. This is *santosa* (contentment) – try to practice it in all areas of life.

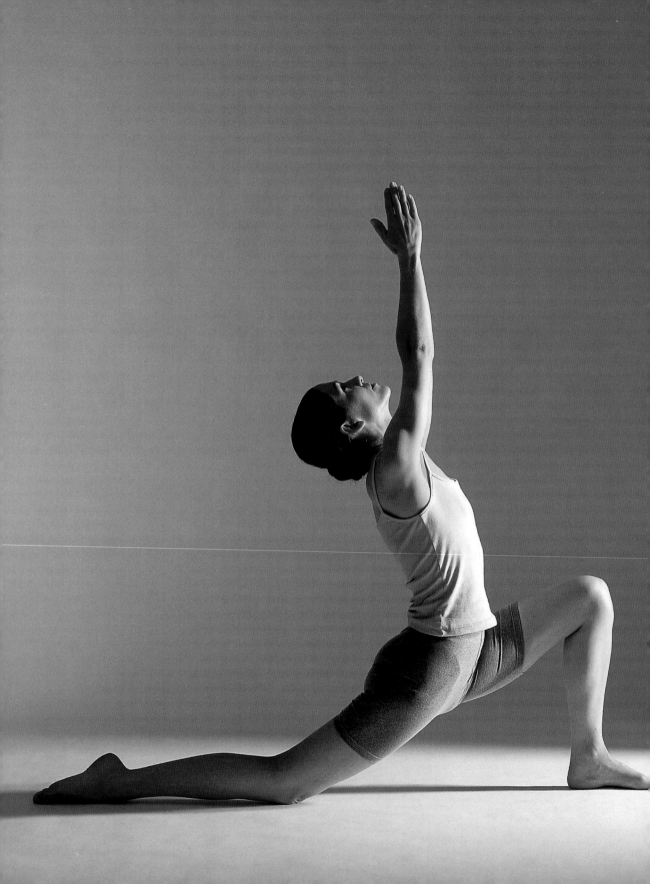

# the postures

The practice of yoga postures (*asana*) brings balance, equilibrium and good health to the body. It is a gentle but powerful way of working not just muscles, tendons and joints, but internal organs too. The postures on the following pages improve digestion, elimination and breathing, and they tone, detoxify and strengthen the body's systems.

The postures in this chapter have been chosen as a broad cross-section of attainable poses that you can practise at home. You may already be familiar with them from attending yoga classes. They will help you to get into a routine of self-practice sessions (see pages 48–9) .

As you practise the postures, your body will yield or resist in various ways. The postures may feel different every day – sometimes easy, sometimes difficult. Don't worry – this is yoga at work, a way of tuning in to or connecting with your inner self.

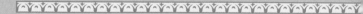

# mountain pose

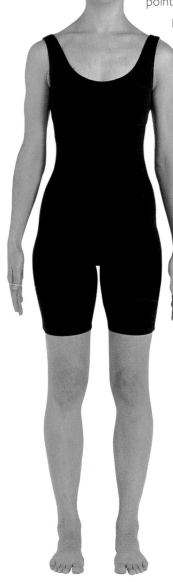

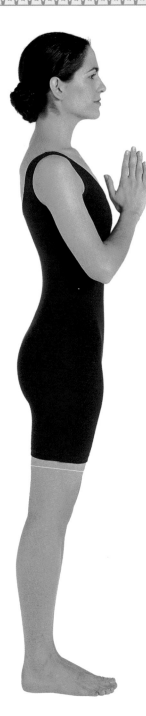

TADASANA Mountain pose promotes calm, stillness and an awareness of your "centre". It embodies a key aspect of *asana* practice in that it teaches you to stand firm without mental or physical wavering. The pose forms the starting point for other standing poses, and it grounds the mind and body in preparation for more complex poses.

### First variation

Stand with your feet parallel and slightly apart. Spread the soles evenly and let them feel rooted to the earth. Softly, lift the entire front of your body and let the back of your body release toward the floor. Extend your fingers gently downward. Keep your head level and your gaze steady. Stand tall. Stay here for 4–8 breaths.

🕉 Let yourself feel connected to the earth – the solid, physical reality of being. Don't rush through this posture.

### Second variation

Stand with your feet together, pressing your big toe joints firmly into the ground. Lift your inner ankles, kneecaps and thighs. Find your centre of balance and bring your hands together at the middle of your chest. Release any tension from your neck and shoulders and, when you feel balanced, gently close your eyes. Stay here for a few breaths.

# standing forward bend

UTTANASANA  Forward bends stimulate the spine, aid digestion and elimination and help to remove toxins from the body. This pose aligns the legs and hips, stretches the hamstrings and tones your whole system by inverting the upper body. Try to fold forward by relaxing your torso rather than pushing down to reach your toes. If you have a stiff back, take this pose gently and pay attention to your breath.

1 Stand in the first variation of mountain pose. Lift your arms over your head on an in-breath. Keep your palms apart and facing each other. Relax your shoulders.

Focus on releasing tension from your tongue and jaw and the soles of your feet.

If you cannot place your hands on the floor, fold forward as in step 2 but bend your knees a little. They should point forward and be directly above your feet. Grasp your elbows with your hands, or let your hands rest on your legs for extra support.

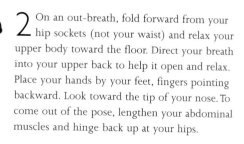

2 On an out-breath, fold forward from your hip sockets (not your waist) and relax your upper body toward the floor. Direct your breath into your upper back to help it open and relax. Place your hands by your feet, fingers pointing backward. Look toward the tip of your nose. To come out of the pose, lengthen your abdominal muscles and hinge back up at your hips.

# triangle

TRIKONASANA  This posture has a strong geometric quality – its Sanskrit name is translated as three (*tri*) angle (*kona*) posture (*asana*). In fact, several triangles are formed by the position of the arms, legs and torso. Triangle helps to align the hips, legs and torso and to develop strength, flexibility and stamina. One of the challenges of the pose is to breathe evenly and steadily. To keep the posture strong but light, try visualizing a huge bird floating on a current of air with its wings outstretched.

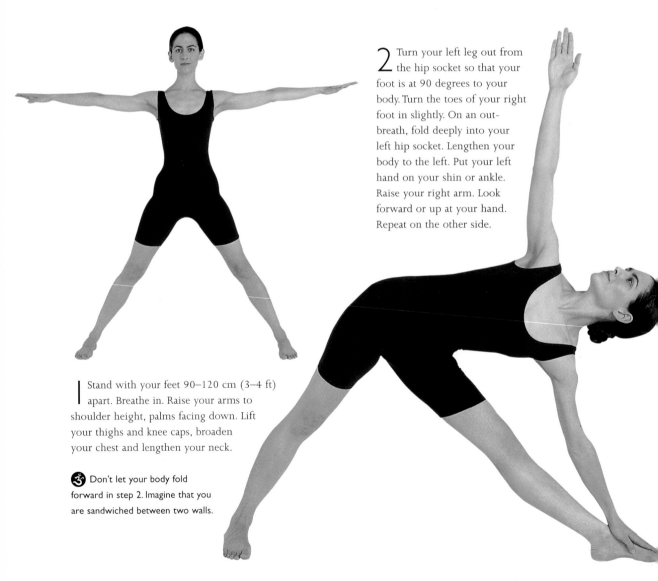

2 Turn your left leg out from the hip socket so that your foot is at 90 degrees to your body. Turn the toes of your right foot in slightly. On an out-breath, fold deeply into your left hip socket. Lengthen your body to the left. Put your left hand on your shin or ankle. Raise your right arm. Look forward or up at your hand. Repeat on the other side.

1 Stand with your feet 90–120 cm (3–4 ft) apart. Breathe in. Raise your arms to shoulder height, palms facing down. Lift your thighs and knee caps, broaden your chest and lengthen your neck.

🕉 Don't let your body fold forward in step 2. Imagine that you are sandwiched between two walls.

# revolved side stretch

PARAVOTTANASANA This gives your hamstrings a powerful stretch and builds an awareness of the relationship between your lower back and your legs, and the way in which muscles in the front of your body can support your back. Revolved side stretch is a humbling posture for most of us – we cannot usually do it as well as we think we should!

1 Stand with your feet 90–120 cm (3–4 ft) apart. Turn your left foot out by 90 degrees and turn in your right foot. On an in-breath, swing your hips round to face over your left leg. Release your tailbone toward the floor and lift your lower abdominals so that your pelvis sits vertically on top of your legs. Lift and straighten your knees and thighs. Breathe in and raise your arms above your head.

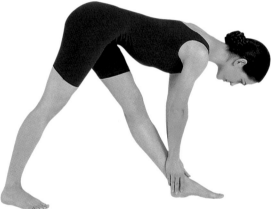

2 On an out-breath softly fold forward from your hip sockets and place your hands on your shin, ankle or the floor – wherever is comfortable. Keep your knees straight and your hips parallel. Lengthen your spine and check that your neck and head are aligned. Lift your abdominals slightly as you lengthen your ribs away from your hips. Breathe. Repeat on the other side.

If your hamstrings are tight, fold forward by 45 degrees instead of 90 degrees. Put your hands on your thighs.

The aim of this posture is the correct alignment of your legs, pelvis and torso. Visualize your kidneys as a pair of weighing scales on your back, keeping you level. Don't twist your torso.

# hands-to-feet pose

PRASARITA PADOTTANASANA   The Sanskrit name of this posture is translated as spread (*prasarita*) foot (*pada*) stretched (*uttan*) posture (*asana*). The pose provides a deep and invigorating stretch for the legs, stimulates the digestive system and helps to clear the mind, as well as focusing your attention on the alignment of your feet, ankles and hips. The key to doing this posture lies in bending from the hip socket rather than the waist. Try to visualize this movement before you do it.

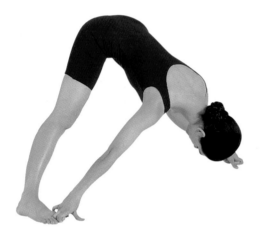

1 Stand with your feet parallel and approximately 135 cm (4½ ft) apart. Breathe in, pull up your thighs and kneecaps and raise your arms in the air. Fold forward at your hip joints keeping your knees and thigh muscles strongly lifted. Bring your hands to your feet and clasp the backs of your ankles or use your index and middle fingers to clasp your big toes – whichever is easier. Breathe in and lengthen your torso, keeping your legs straight and your neck in line with your spine. Pull up your abdominal and pelvic floor muscles for support. Open your chest wide. Breathe evenly.

If you find this posture difficult, are stiff or have a back injury, do it with your hands on the fronts of your thighs and your knees slightly bent. Keep your spine in a straight line.

2 On an out-breath rotate a little further forward at the hips (even by a few degrees), keeping your spine and legs straight. Direct your breath into the area of the stretch. Lift your elbows up toward the ceiling and ease your chest down toward the floor. Do not bend your knees.

If you find this posture easy, do it with your legs a little closer together and aim to gently lower the crown of your head to the floor in between your feet.

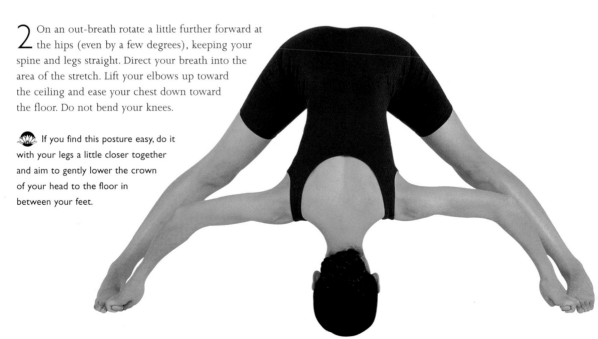

# extended-angle pose

PARSVAKONASANA  Regular practice of this posture brings flexibility and strength to the spine and legs, and improves digestion, elimination, breathing and an awareness of body alignment. If you find the triangle (see page 56) tough on your lower back, you may find this posture easier. Consider the way the side of the body opens up – let the heart centre be free. Feel rooted into the ground at your back heel and enjoy the expansiveness of the pose with confidence.

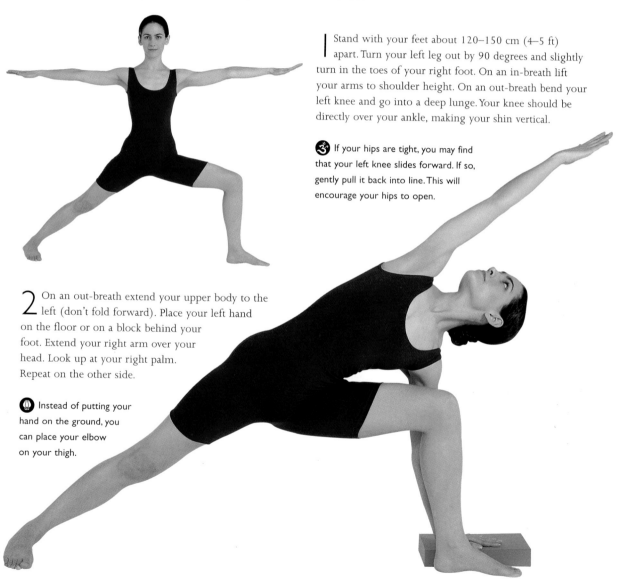

1 Stand with your feet about 120–150 cm (4–5 ft) apart. Turn your left leg out by 90 degrees and slightly turn in the toes of your right foot. On an in-breath lift your arms to shoulder height. On an out-breath bend your left knee and go into a deep lunge. Your knee should be directly over your ankle, making your shin vertical.

🕉 If your hips are tight, you may find that your left knee slides forward. If so, gently pull it back into line. This will encourage your hips to open.

2 On an out-breath extend your upper body to the left (don't fold forward). Place your left hand on the floor or on a block behind your foot. Extend your right arm over your head. Look up at your right palm. Repeat on the other side.

☸ Instead of putting your hand on the ground, you can place your elbow on your thigh.

# warrior poses

VIRABHADRASANA These two bold and dynamic postures are named after Virabhadra, a warrior of Indian mythology. Both postures work strongly on the connection between the hips, pelvis and lower back, the seats of the lowest three *chakras*. They tone and strengthen the thigh muscles and harness energy and strength which are directed wherever they are needed in the body or mind.

**First variation**

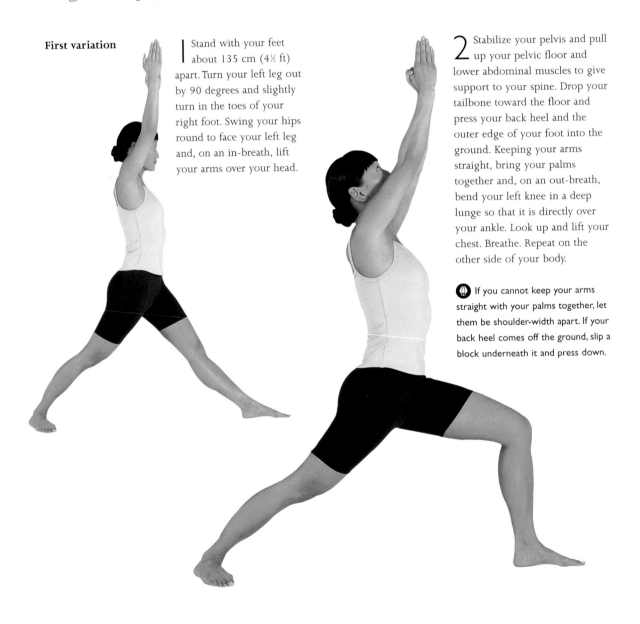

1 Stand with your feet about 135 cm (4½ ft) apart. Turn your left leg out by 90 degrees and slightly turn in the toes of your right foot. Swing your hips round to face your left leg and, on an in-breath, lift your arms over your head.

2 Stabilize your pelvis and pull up your pelvic floor and lower abdominal muscles to give support to your spine. Drop your tailbone toward the floor and press your back heel and the outer edge of your foot into the ground. Keeping your arms straight, bring your palms together and, on an out-breath, bend your left knee in a deep lunge so that it is directly over your ankle. Look up and lift your chest. Breathe. Repeat on the other side of your body.

If you cannot keep your arms straight with your palms together, let them be shoulder-width apart. If your back heel comes off the ground, slip a block underneath it and press down.

**Second variation**

Stand with your feet about 135 cm (4½ ft) apart. Turn your left leg out by 90 degrees and slightly turn in the toes of your right foot. On an in-breath lift your arms to shoulder height and lengthen your torso. Pull up your pelvic floor and lower abdominal muscles.

**3** You can make a dynamic sequence of these two steps. Breathe out and go into step two, breathe in and go back into step one. Repeat this a few times and listen to the quality of your breath as you do so.

**!** Both variations can hurt your knees if you do them incorrectly. Make sure your knee always faces the same direction as your foot – don't let it collapse inward. Lift the thighs in step 1 of both variations. When you go into a deep lunge, keep your front knee directly above your ankle, your shin perpendicular and your thigh parallel to the floor.

2 On an out-breath, turn your head to gaze along the middle finger of your left hand. Bend your left knee in a deep lunge. Breathe. Repeat on the other side of your body.

# down-facing dog

ADHO MUKHA SVANASANA  The aptly named down-facing dog posture really does resemble a dog stretching. It is an energizing and refreshing pose that develops great strength and freedom of movement in your upper body. If you are a beginner, you may at first find the posture tough on the wrists. Take as many rests as you need, but try to persevere – the results can be dramatic.

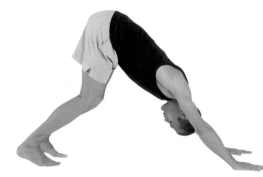

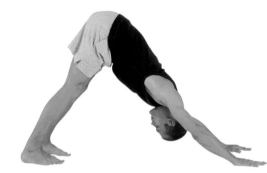

I Begin on all fours with your hands shoulder-width apart on the floor, fingers spread with middle fingers pointing forward. Tuck your toes underneath you and lift your hips high in the air. Your feet should be hip-width apart, your knees bent and your heels off the ground. Pull your shoulder blades back toward your waist. Keep your armpits open. Take a few breaths.

2 Pull your lower abdominals up toward your spine. Tilt your tailbone to the ceiling and press your pubic bone back between your legs. Press firmly down through your hands and, on an out-breath, pull up your thigh muscles and straighten your legs – don't let your lower back curve. Stretch your heels down to the floor, relax your neck and look at the tip of your nose. Take at least five breaths.

A variation of this pose is called the giraffe pose. When you are in step 2 of down-facing dog, bring your hands a little closer to your feet and then walk your left hand and your left foot about 10–15 cm (4–6 in) forward. Keep your legs straight, your thighs and abdominal muscles lifted, and your tailbone high. This should produce a powerful stretch in your left leg and along your left side. Return to step 2 of down-facing dog and repeat with your right hand and your right foot.

# up-facing dog

URDHVA MUKHA SVANASANA This invigorating posture stimulates the nervous system. It requires strong wrists and spinal flexibility – as with down-facing dog, these things come rapidly with regular practice. Up-facing dog is a powerful backbend – if it causes discomfort in your lower back, concentrate on pulling up your abdominal muscles to give maximum support to your spine. Alternatively, practise the easier modification (see box, below) until you have more flexibility. You can flow down-facing dog and up-facing dog together in a short sequence.

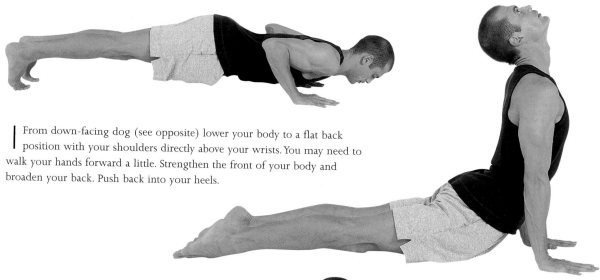

1 From down-facing dog (see opposite) lower your body to a flat back position with your shoulders directly above your wrists. You may need to walk your hands forward a little. Strengthen the front of your body and broaden your back. Push back into your heels.

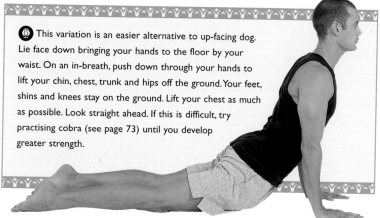

This variation is an easier alternative to up-facing dog. Lie face down bringing your hands to the floor by your waist. On an in-breath, push down through your hands to lift your chin, chest, trunk and hips off the ground. Your feet, shins and knees stay on the ground. Lift your chest as much as possible. Look straight ahead. If this is difficult, try practising cobra (see page 73) until you develop greater strength.

2 On an in-breath, move your whole body forward and upward. Roll forward onto the tops of your feet and point your toes. Raise the centre of your chest skyward and look up. Strongly lift the front of your body and your thigh muscles. Keep your neck long and don't let your shoulders collapse. Breathe.

# tree pose

VRKSASANA  Tree pose, like all balancing postures, helps to develop and maintain physical and mental equilibrium. Balance is strongly affected by your emotional state and, by learning to balance the body, you can learn how to calm the mind. Visualize a single magnificent tree rooting down into the earth and growing up toward the sun.

1 Begin in the first variation of mountain pose (see page 54). Make sure that your weight is evenly balanced between both feet.

2 Transfer your weight onto your left foot and raise your right knee to your chest. Clasp it with your hands. Feel your lower back lengthen and your abdominal muscles engage.

🪷 If you feel comfortable and balanced in step 3, try the final posture. Stretch your arms over your head, keeping your neck and shoulders relaxed. Stay here for a few breaths. Consider the way in which a tree is both strong and flexible – how it is firmly rooted yet can bend and blow in the wind. Make sure that you are not rigid – let go of any tension in your feet, shoulders, tongue and face. If you find this easy, bring the palms of your hands together, keeping your elbows straight, and take a few breaths with your eyes closed.

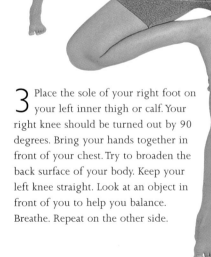

3 Place the sole of your right foot on your left inner thigh or calf. Your right knee should be turned out by 90 degrees. Bring your hands together in front of your chest. Try to broaden the back surface of your body. Keep your left knee straight. Look at an object in front of you to help you balance. Breathe. Repeat on the other side.

# eagle pose

GARUDASANA  Eagle pose turns your attention inward by focusing energy at *ajna chakra* (see page 25), which lies above and between your eyes. The posture gives a strong stretch to the muscles across your shoulders and upper back, helping to release tension in these areas. The pose is useful if you spend a lot of time working in a fixed position at a keyboard.

🕉 The eagle symbolizes the triumph of the spirit over the intellect. When we find our balance in this posture we can gaze through the third eye (*ajna chakra*) and bring our true nature into sharp focus.

Stand with your feet a little way apart. On an in-breath raise your arms to shoulder height. On an out-breath bend both knees as low as possible without lifting your heels from the ground. Cross your left leg over your right, tucking your left foot behind your right calf if you can. Keep your legs bent low and your hips level. On an out-breath cross your right arm over your left with your palms facing up. Bend your elbows and bring your hands together so that you hold your right thumb with your left hand. Lift your elbows. Breathe steadily allowing the space between your shoulders to expand. Close your eyes and focus on *ajna chakra*. Repeat the posture crossing your arms and legs the opposite way.

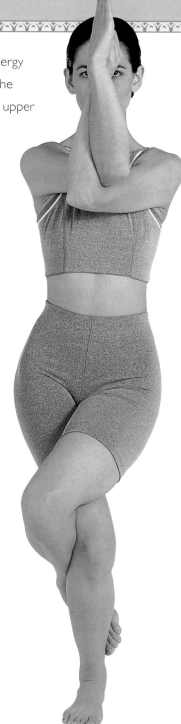

🪷 The leg posture for eagle pose requires strong knees. If you have a knee injury or this posture feels uncomfortable in your knees, or even if you find it difficult to balance, practise only the arm position. Cross your right arm over your left (as shown), bend your elbows and bring your palms together. Extend the stretch across your back by raising your elbows to shoulder height.

🕉 As with many asymmetrical postures in yoga, you may find this pose easier on one side of the body. With each practise, alternate the arm that is uppermost until you are equally flexible on both sides.

# crescent-moon pose

ARDHA CHANDRASANA  The short series of movements that create crescent-moon pose build strength in the upper and lower back, thighs and abdominal muscles. The series helps to open and expand the chest *chakra* (*anahata*), which is the centre of ambition, hope, love and compassion. Like all backbends, crescent-moon pose has an energizing and rejuvenating effect on the body. It also forms part of the sun salutation sequence (see page 100).

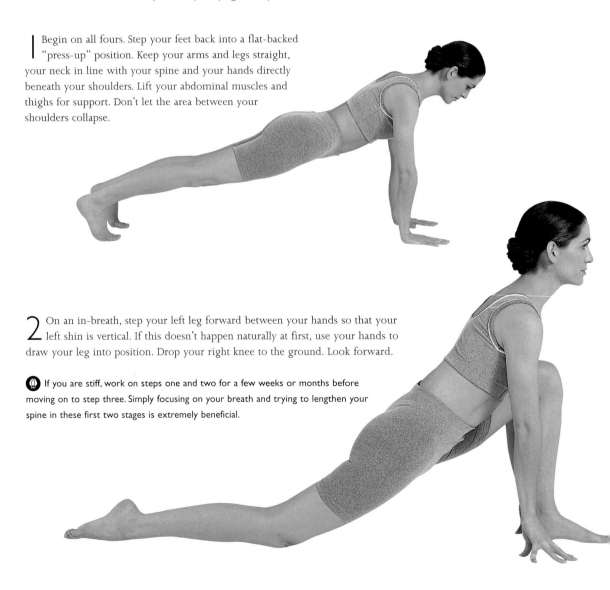

1 Begin on all fours. Step your feet back into a flat-backed "press-up" position. Keep your arms and legs straight, your neck in line with your spine and your hands directly beneath your shoulders. Lift your abdominal muscles and thighs for support. Don't let the area between your shoulders collapse.

2 On an in-breath, step your left leg forward between your hands so that your left shin is vertical. If this doesn't happen naturally at first, use your hands to draw your leg into position. Drop your right knee to the ground. Look forward.

🌑 If you are stiff, work on steps one and two for a few weeks or months before moving on to step three. Simply focusing on your breath and trying to lengthen your spine in these first two stages is extremely beneficial.

3 As you breathe out let your inner thigh muscles relax and then lift your abdominal muscles to support your spine. Breathe in, raise your upper body and rest your hands on your left knee. Broaden your chest and drop your tailbone. Breathe. Repeat on the other side.

❗ If this posture hurts your knees, check the alignment of your front leg – your knee should be directly above your ankle, rather than overshooting it. If it still hurts, practise another backbend, such as cobra (see page 73) or bridge pose (see page 77).

🌸 If you feel comfortable in step 3, move into the final pose. On an in-breath lift your arms over your head. Keep your abdominal muscles strongly drawn up to give maximum support to your spine. Let your chest – the seat of the heart *chakra* – open and expand. Allow your chest to move upward and your head to drop back a little way. Look up and concentrate on breathing steadily.

If you feel comfortable and balanced, bring the palms of your hands together while keeping your arms straight. Breathe. On an out-breath take your hands to the ground and step the left leg back to join the right. Repeat the pose with the opposite leg.

🕉 Although crescent-moon pose is a backbend, like all backbends it is also a front stretch. Sometimes during backbends there is a tendency to crumple the spine into itself in an effort to attain the posture. In fact, what you should be doing is stretching and lengthening the spine in order to create as much space between the vertebrae as possible. You can do this by lifting and lengthening the muscle structures in the front of the body, using them as spinal stabilizers. When you do crescent-moon pose, try to concentrate on the front of your body and you will find that the backbend will follow naturally in its own time.

# child pose

BALASANA This lovely nurturing posture resembles the curled up position of a baby in the womb. Child pose is soothing for the back and restful for the head, face and eyes; it also develops softness and flexibility in the ankles, knees and hips. As you breathe in and out in child pose, try to become aware of your head and pelvis as two heavy weights releasing toward the floor and gently stretching the spine between them. Child pose can flow smoothly into camel pose (see opposite).

1 Kneel with your knees and ankles close together (don't sit back on your heels yet). On an in-breath, lift your arms gently above your head and feel your whole back lengthen. Keep your neck and low back long and loose. Breathe steadily.

2 On an out-breath, sit back on your heels and gently fold forward. Lower your forehead to the floor and rest your hands alongside your feet, palms facing upward. Breathe softly and steadily. Relax the muscles in your neck, shoulders and chest.

If you find kneeling uncomfortable, try placing a rolled up mat or blanket under your ankles to take the pressure off the tops of your feet. You can place a block between your hips and heels if your knees feel tight, or rest your forehead on a block if your head does not easily reach the floor.

Observe your breathing through the movement of your diaphragm pressed against your thighs.

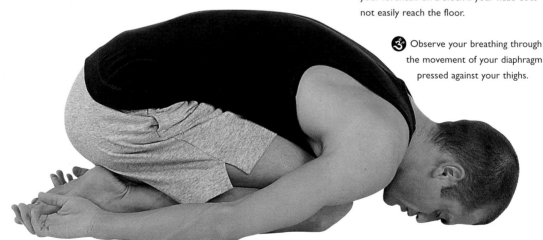

# camel pose

USTRASANA This is a strong but secure backbend that tones the muscles in the thighs, abdomen, neck and back and stimulates the thyroid gland. It promotes deep breathing and releases tightness in the chest and throat. Avoid it if you have a neck or back injury, are pregnant, have had recent abdominal surgery, or if the pose causes nausea or dizziness.

1 Kneel with your knees hip-width apart. On an in-breath, stretch your arms over your head. Let the fronts of your thighs lengthen and your lower back release. Pull up your lower abdominal and pelvic floor muscles. On an out-breath, drop your right hand to your right heel.

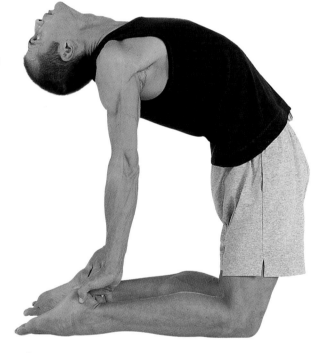

2 With your right hand on your right heel, lift upward through the fronts of your thighs and your abdomen and left arm. Look down toward your right heel. Your buttock muscles will automatically contract. Return to kneeling upright and repeat steps 1 and 2 with your left arm.

3 Kneel upright and this time take both hands back to grasp your heels. Press forward through your thighs, open your chest, lift the front of your body, elongate your spine and let your head drop gently back toward the earth.

If you cannot reach your heels in camel pose, tuck your toes underneath to raise your heels slightly.

Try to visualize yourself forming an arc, like a rainbow.

# cow-face pose

**GOMUKASANA** This curiously named posture is said to look like the shape of a cow's head (the feet are the cow's horns). Although the posture appears very knotted, it is a wonderful way to release upper back and shoulder tension and free the area around the sacrum, buttocks and thighs. Try to focus on expanding your body within the posture.

🕉 If this posture hurts your knees or you find it difficult to get both knees into position, start by practising with one leg only. Sit with your left leg stretched out in front, bend your right knee and bring your right calf over your left leg. Try to align your two knees. Swap legs.

🕉 If your hands don't meet behind your back, dangle a belt or strap from the upper hand and catch it with the lower hand.

🕉 If you find it difficult to achieve the leg position, just concentrate on doing the arm part of the posture while kneeling, or sitting on a low stool or chair.

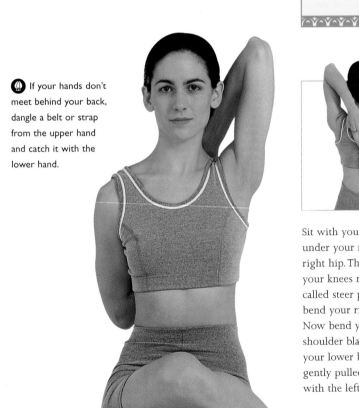

Sit with your legs out in front of you. Bend your left leg under your right and place your left ankle beside your right hip. Then bend your right leg over your left so that your knees rest one above the other, ankles relaxed (this is called steer pose). Raise your left arm over your head and bend your right arm behind your back, palm facing out. Now bend your left arm so that your palm faces your shoulder blades. Clasp your hands together. Check that your lower back is not arching and your abdominals are gently pulled in. Keep your head centred. Repeat the pose with the left leg and right arm uppermost.

# sitting leg stretch

PARIVRTTA JANU SIRSASANA  In this strong side stretch, the kidneys, liver, spleen and lower back muscles receive a thorough workout. Sitting leg stretch also has great detoxifying effects. Even if you are stiff at first, approach this posture carefully and methodically – you will soon feel the benefits.

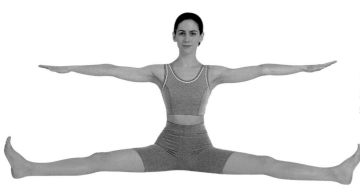

1 Sit with your legs as wide apart as you can comfortably manage with a straight spine. Your toes and kneecaps face directly upward. Lift your lower abdominal muscles and, on an in-breath, lift your arms up to shoulder height.

🏵 If you find it difficult to sit up straight in this position, sit on the edge of a block.

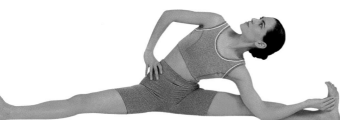

2 On an out-breath, fold your body to the left. Keep your chest facing forward and both hips on the floor. Put your left hand on your foot or on the floor inside your leg. Put your right hand on your right hip. Breathe in. Look up beyond your right shoulder. Repeat on the other side.

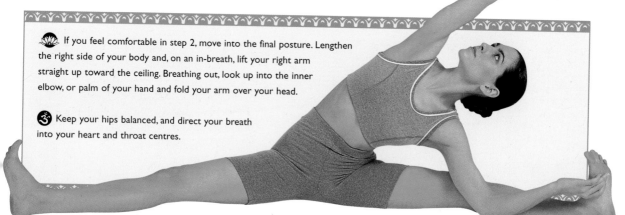

🏵 If you feel comfortable in step 2, move into the final posture. Lengthen the right side of your body and, on an in-breath, lift your right arm straight up toward the ceiling. Breathing out, look up into the inner elbow, or palm of your hand and fold your arm over your head.

🕉 Keep your hips balanced, and direct your breath into your heart and throat centres.

# sitting forward bend

PASCHMOTTANASANA  Many people find this posture frustrating – perhaps because we believe that we should be able to bend flat if we try hard enough. In fact, because we sit on chairs from an early age, we lose a great deal of flexibility in our lower back and legs. The keys to this posture are patience and practice rather than brute force.

1 Sit on the floor and stretch out your legs, pushing the insides of your heels and your big toe joints forward to keep your inner legs extended. On an in-breath, raise your arms above your head. Lift your abdominal muscles.

2 Fold forward from your hips on an out-breath. Extend the spine as far as you can (don't lead with your chin). Rest your hands on your legs. Align your head and spine. Keep your chest area open.

Unless you are very flexible, sit on a block to make the pose much easier. Alternatively, bend your knees, hold the soles of your feet and bring your chest to your thighs – now gradually extend your legs. Another modification is to practise with straight legs while holding onto a belt that is looped around your feet.

3 Gently clasp your toes, ankles or whichever part of your legs you can reach. On an in-breath, lift your body and your abdominal and pelvic floor muscles and lengthen your spine. On your next out-breath fold softly forward, bending your elbows outward and keeping your neck and shoulders relaxed. Repeat for several breaths.

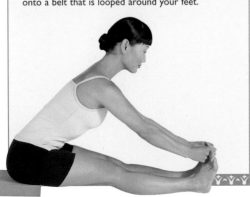

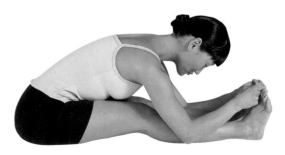

# cobra

BHUJANGASANA  The shape of this posture resembles a snake that is ready to strike. It helps to develop strength and flexibility in the upper spine, tones the digestive, eliminative, nervous and respiratory systems, and like all backbends, stimulates the brain and is generally refreshing and invigorating. Child pose (see page 68) is an excellent resting position after cobra.

1 Lie face down, relax your heels and gently lift your abdominal muscles. Place your hands on the ground beneath your shoulders. On an in-breath raise your chest, head and hands from the ground using the strength of your abdomen and back.

🕉 This posture should be full of potential energy. Visualize a cobra drawing back its head to strike.

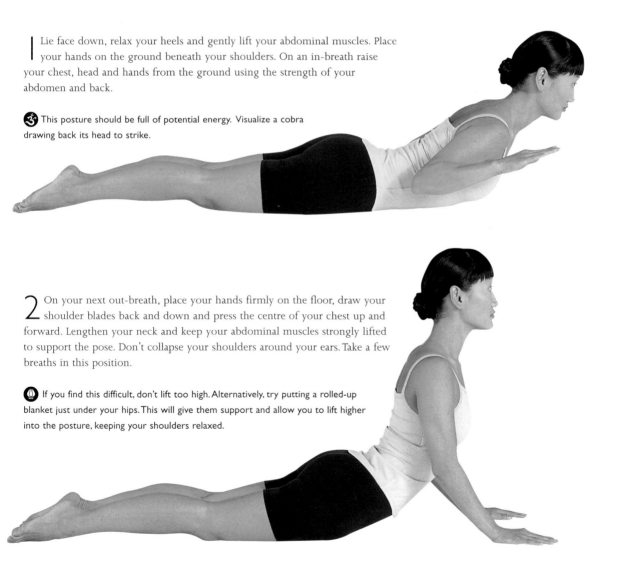

2 On your next out-breath, place your hands firmly on the floor, draw your shoulder blades back and down and press the centre of your chest up and forward. Lengthen your neck and keep your abdominal muscles strongly lifted to support the pose. Don't collapse your shoulders around your ears. Take a few breaths in this position.

🪷 If you find this difficult, don't lift too high. Alternatively, try putting a rolled-up blanket just under your hips. This will give them support and allow you to lift higher into the posture, keeping your shoulders relaxed.

# tailor pose

BADDHA KONASANA  The Sanskrit name for this pose is translated as bound (*baddha*) angle (*kona*) posture (*asana*). The angle referred to is that between the legs and torso. The body folds gently forward at the hips, which helps to develop hip flexibility and spinal extension. Tailor pose strengthens the lower abdomen and helps to relieve menstrual and bladder problems, including period pain.

1  Sit with the soles of your feet together and your back straight. Pull up your lower abdominal muscles to give support to your spine. Place your hands on your feet, ankles or shins, wherever they will comfortably reach. Allow your inner thighs to relax and let your knees drop to the sides. Breathe in and broaden and lift your chest.

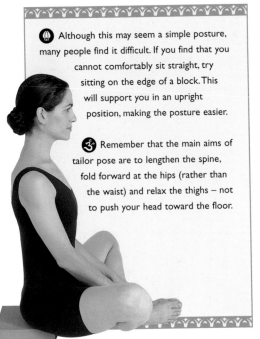

🛇 Although this may seem a simple posture, many people find it difficult. If you find that you cannot comfortably sit straight, try sitting on the edge of a block. This will support you in an upright position, making the posture easier.

🕉 Remember that the main aims of tailor pose are to lengthen the spine, fold forward at the hips (rather than the waist) and relax the thighs – not to push your head toward the floor.

2  As you breathe out, keep your chest broad and fold softly forward at your hips. Keep your back flat. When you can go no further, allow your head to drop gently and your spine to curve. Don't hunch your shoulders or pull on your feet. Relax. Breathe out to release your thighs and breathe in to lengthen your spine. Come up slowly.

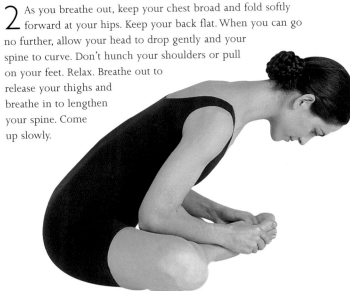

# half-lotus

PADMASANA  The half-lotus and lotus are traditional meditation postures, and ones that many people readily associate with yoga. Half-lotus requires flexibility in your hips but, with practice, it should be attainable for most people. Enhance your experience of the posture by letting your head "rise" and your spine "grow". Visualize a lotus flower floating on water.

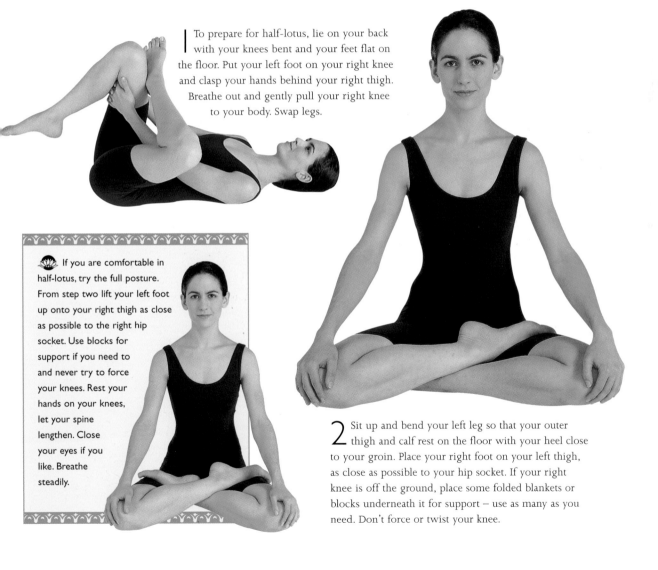

1 To prepare for half-lotus, lie on your back with your knees bent and your feet flat on the floor. Put your left foot on your right knee and clasp your hands behind your right thigh. Breathe out and gently pull your right knee to your body. Swap legs.

If you are comfortable in half-lotus, try the full posture. From step two lift your left foot up onto your right thigh as close as possible to the right hip socket. Use blocks for support if you need to and never try to force your knees. Rest your hands on your knees, let your spine lengthen. Close your eyes if you like. Breathe steadily.

2 Sit up and bend your left leg so that your outer thigh and calf rest on the floor with your heel close to your groin. Place your right foot on your left thigh, as close as possible to your hip socket. If your right knee is off the ground, place some folded blankets or blocks underneath it for support – use as many as you need. Don't force or twist your knee.

# knees-to-chest pose

APANASANA  This simple pose is a wonderful way to relax the large muscles in the lower back and reduce tension in the area of the sacrum and hips. It is also an excellent counterpose for backbends or twisting postures. Take your time in this posture and try to visualize the back surface of your body slowly spreading out, softening and loosening. Observe how the simple act of breathing in can expand the muscles in the back of your body and how breathing out releases them.

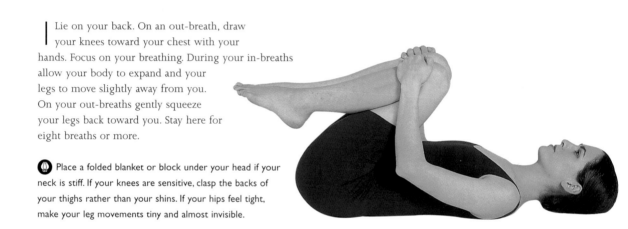

1 Lie on your back. On an out-breath, draw your knees toward your chest with your hands. Focus on your breathing. During your in-breaths allow your body to expand and your legs to move slightly away from you. On your out-breaths gently squeeze your legs back toward you. Stay here for eight breaths or more.

🔅 Place a folded blanket or block under your head if your neck is stiff. If your knees are sensitive, clasp the backs of your thighs rather than your shins. If your hips feel tight, make your leg movements tiny and almost invisible.

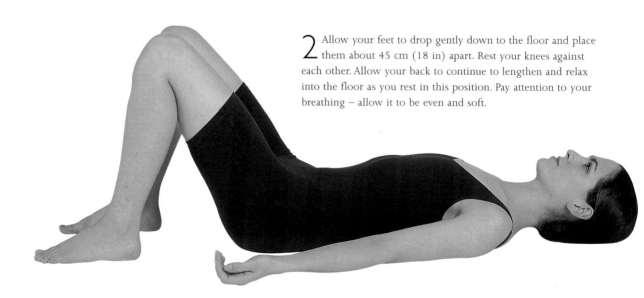

2 Allow your feet to drop gently down to the floor and place them about 45 cm (18 in) apart. Rest your knees against each other. Allow your back to continue to lengthen and relax into the floor as you rest in this position. Pay attention to your breathing – allow it to be even and soft.

# bridge pose

SETU BANDHASANA  Bridge pose is a safe and strong backbend that is excellent for beginners. The pose helps to develop flexibility, strength and an awareness of the way in which you can use your abdominal and pelvic floor muscles (*mula* and *uddiyana bandhas*; see page 107). Bridge pose strengthens your legs and helps your chest to open out, which in turn frees the heart centre (*anahata*). It also stimulates the spine and the glands in the neck, and prepares the body for shoulderstand (see page 86).

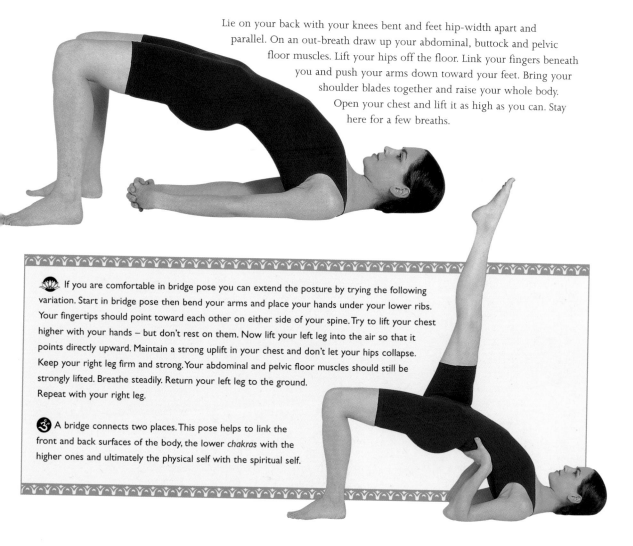

Lie on your back with your knees bent and feet hip-width apart and parallel. On an out-breath draw up your abdominal, buttock and pelvic floor muscles. Lift your hips off the floor. Link your fingers beneath you and push your arms down toward your feet. Bring your shoulder blades together and raise your whole body. Open your chest and lift it as high as you can. Stay here for a few breaths.

If you are comfortable in bridge pose you can extend the posture by trying the following variation. Start in bridge pose then bend your arms and place your hands under your lower ribs. Your fingertips should point toward each other on either side of your spine. Try to lift your chest higher with your hands – but don't rest on them. Now lift your left leg into the air so that it points directly upward. Maintain a strong uplift in your chest and don't let your hips collapse. Keep your right leg firm and strong. Your abdominal and pelvic floor muscles should still be strongly lifted. Breathe steadily. Return your left leg to the ground. Repeat with your right leg.

A bridge connects two places. This pose helps to link the front and back surfaces of the body, the lower *chakras* with the higher ones and ultimately the physical self with the spiritual self.

# three twists

Twisting postures increase suppleness in your spine and strongly stimulate your internal organs – in particular, your kidneys, stomach, pancreas and spleen. They also help you to develop an awareness of your breathing. There are many variations of twisting postures in yoga – some, such as the lying-down twist shown here (twist A), are passive and rely on the weight of the body to create the twist; others, such as the sitting twists (B and C), are more active.

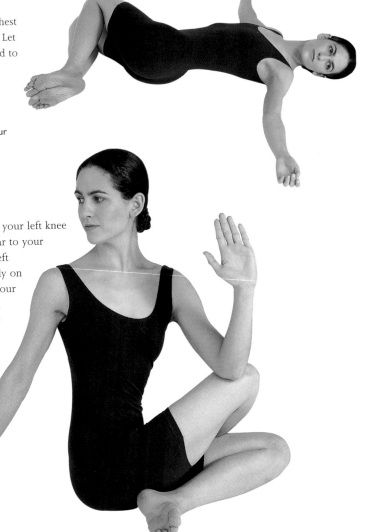

**Twist A**

Lie on your back, bring your knees to your chest and spread your arms out at shoulder height. Let your knees fall to one side and turn your head to the other. Stay here for 8–12 breaths. Release any tension from your feet, face, hands and inner thighs. Repeat on the other side.

If this makes you feel uncomfortable, move your knees away from your body to reduce the strain.

**Twist B**

Sit with your legs straight out in front. Bend your left knee so that your left foot rests on the ground near to your right thigh. Bring your right leg over your left thigh and rest the sole of your right foot fully on the floor. Lengthen your spine and pull up your lower abdominal muscles. On an out-breath, rotate your body to the right and place your left hand on your right knee. Draw your navel in toward your spine and, on an out-breath, rotate your body further. Place your left elbow on the outer side of your right knee. Place your right hand lightly on the floor to give you balance (don't collapse all your weight onto this hand). Breathe steadily in this position, trying to increase the twist on each out-breath.

**Twist C** is more challenging than the previous two postures. The knee is held by the arms, which helps to promote a strong twist in the trunk. It is important – in this and similar poses – to extend the twist throughout the whole body, from the base of the spine to the top of the head. (A common mistake is to do the twist with the chin rather than the body!) Also try to release tension from the muscles of the jaw, tongue and face (there is a tendency to clench these areas) during the posture. Let your head feel as though it's floating lightly on the top of your spine.

| Sit with your legs out in front. Bend your left leg and draw the foot toward you. Keep your right leg straight. Breathe in, lift your left arm over your head and lengthen your spine.

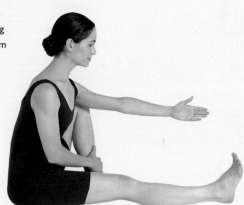

2 Draw up your abdominal muscles. Bend forward on an out-breath bringing your left arm down inside your left leg to reach toward your right foot. Drop your left shoulder onto the inside of your left knee.

3 Turn your left palm outward and, leaning forward, bend your left elbow and fold it around your left shin. Take your right hand behind your back and link your hands, or take hold of your right wrist with your left hand. Lift your chest, rotate your entire body and look back over your right shoulder.

Sit on a block or folded blanket to raise your hips if you need to. You can also use a belt to link your hands.

# pigeon pose

KAPOTASANA  The muscle structures in the hips, thighs and lower back are closely integrated and this backbending posture utilizes all of them. Pigeon pose can produce excellent flexibility in your hip joints and a strong stretch in your buttocks and the backs of your thighs. The first stage of the pose alone provides an intense, passive stretch in these areas.

1 Kneel on all fours. Bring your left knee forward and your left foot across your right leg to rest on the floor. Slide your right leg back until it is straight (the shin should be flat on the floor). Lower your upper body to rest on your elbows or forehead. Keep your weight centred – don't lean toward the left hip. Breathe.

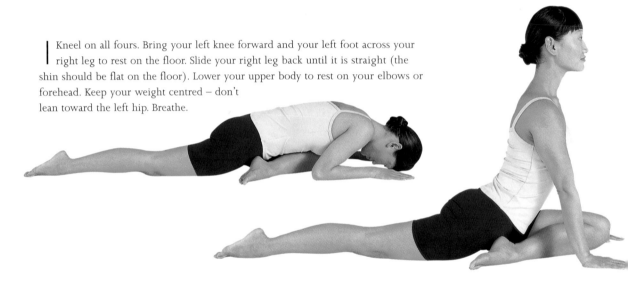

When you feel comfortable in step two, you can try the final posture. Walk your hands back a little farther from their position in step two. Keep lifting your chest and drawing up your abdominal muscles. Try to relax your thighs. Bend your right knee and lift your hands off the floor to balance. Now take hold of your right foot with both hands and fully open your chest. Breathe evenly and steadily.

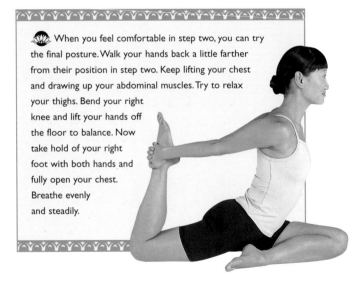

2 Draw your pelvic floor and lower abdominal muscles up toward your spine. Push yourself up with your hands. As you do this, try to keep your inner thighs relaxed and long. Take an in-breath and press your chest up and straighten your arms as much as possible. Keep your shoulders relaxed and open. Direct your breath into the centre of your chest.

Strongly lift the front of your body to alleviate any discomfort in your lower back.

# reclining hero pose

SUPTA VIRASANA  This posture produces an intense stretch in the thighs and is especially useful for people who have tight thigh muscles from running or playing sport. The knees also benefit by becoming stronger, although you should always make sure they are correctly positioned – never let them lift off the floor.

1 Sit on a block, roll your calf muscles slightly outward with your hands and kneel with your hips between your heels, the soles of your feet facing up and your knees close. Rest your hands on your thighs. Lengthen your spine. Breathe steadily.

Sit on as many blocks or books as necessary to ease this posture. Put them between your feet so that your hips just balance on the edge when you sit back.

There is a serene strength in this posture. If you find it comfortable, it is ideal for meditation. You can help to draw your attention inward by lowering your head to your chest and closing your eyes (keep your chest lifted and your back straight).

2 Place your hands on the floor behind you, and gently tilt your pelvis forward, tucking your buttocks underneath and stretching your thighs. (If your knees hurt, stop here.) Lower your elbows onto the floor. Keep lengthening your body and stretching your thighs. Your inner thighs move up and outward.

You need to be quite flexible to practise the final posture, which is done without blocks. Gently lower your body to the floor. Breathing in, take your arms over your head and relax them on the floor behind you. Keep tilting your pelvis in order to minimize the curve in your lower back and maximize the stretch in your thighs. Don't let your knees splay apart. Breathe for a while in this position. To come back up, place your hands on the floor under the small of your back and push down.

If this hurts, stop and consult a teacher about correct alignment.

# wheel

CHAKRASANA This splendid backbend radiates energy through all the *chakras*. Wheel expands the chest and gives strength and flexibility to the entire upper body. The posture requires practice, but your efforts to master it will be rewarded with a wonderful feeling of vibrancy and confidence. Make sure that your muscles are fully warmed up before you do this posture.

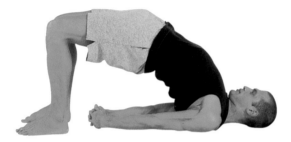

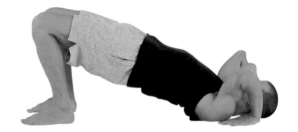

1 Lie on your back with your knees bent and your feet hip-width apart. Move into bridge pose (see page 77).

🕉 It helps to open your chest as fully as you can in preparation for step 3. Try bringing your hands to the back of your lower ribs and lifting your chest as fully as possible. Keep your knees parallel.

2 Bring your hands to the ground beside your head. Your fingertips should face your shoulders and your elbows should point straight upward – don't let them flop sideways. Try to keep your thumbs in contact with the ground. Keep your hips lifted.

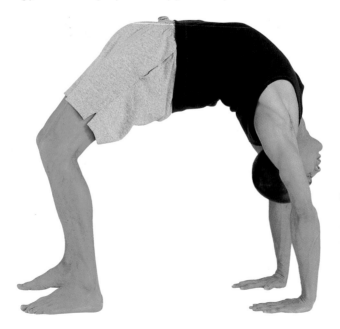

3 Breathe in and lift your body up by pressing down into your hands and feet, and forward through your thighs. Once fully in the posture you can rock forward and backward (toward your toes and then your nose) a few times to open your chest. Return to the ground gently and lie flat for a few moments. Rest in child pose (see page 68).

🔆 If you find step three difficult, remain in step 2 but push up so that the top of your head rests on the floor for a few seconds – don't take much weight on your head. You can also practise camel pose (see page 69) to prepare for this backbend.

# crow

BAKASANA  This posture is said to resemble a crow. Practising it strengthens your upper body, arms and wrists by taking your whole body weight onto your hands. Many people are afraid of falling forward in the pose, but if you can stay in down-facing dog (see page 62) for 10–15 breaths, then you are probably strong enough to hold this posture. You may even find crow easier than it looks!

1 Start in a squatting position with your knees, ankles and hips slightly turned out. Press your elbows gently into your inner knees and bring your palms together in the middle of your chest. Extend your spine and lift your chest. Take a few breaths.

2 Place your hands flat on the floor in front of you. They should be slightly turned in toward each other. Keep your hands flat and lift your knees up so that they are level with your shoulders. You will need to be on tiptoes to do this. Let your arms bend slightly and your elbows point outward.

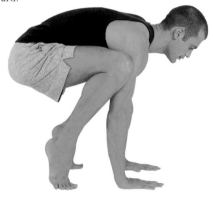

3 Place your inner knees on to the upper part of your arms and gently rock your weight forward. Gaze ahead rather than down at your hands. Transfer your weight smoothly from your feet onto your hands. Balance. Breathe. Come down slowly, with control.

🕉 Don't jump into this posture; move slowly to transfer the weight from your feet to your hands. Trust yourself to find your balance.

# headstand

SIRSASANA Often referred to as the king of postures, the headstand benefits the entire body. It is the ultimate anti-gravity posture, and inverting yourself has a tonic effect on body systems and is even said to slow down the aging process. The headstand rests the heart, stimulates the brain and the nervous system, and develops calm and equilibrium. Avoid headstand during menstruation or if you have a neck injury or a weak or tight back – if in doubt, seek the advice of a yoga teacher.

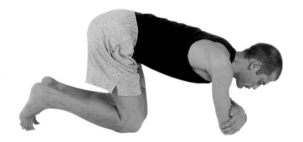

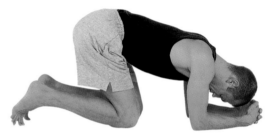

1 Begin on all fours with your toes tucked under. Place your forearms on the ground and grasp the opposite elbow with each hand. This is the ideal distance for your elbows – they should remain in this position for the rest of the posture; don't let them slide apart.

2 Now pivot your hands away from your elbows until one hand can clasp the other. Interlink your fingers. Feel the sides of both hands firmly on the floor.

3 Lift your hips into the air. Draw your shoulders down your back toward your waist, broaden your chest and straighten your legs. Place your head gently in the cradle of your hands.

🛈 You may find it easier to practise headstand in a corner of the room. The walls will stop you falling to one side or letting your elbows separate too far. However, if you use a wall, don't lean against it, just use it to give you a sense of confidence. If you feel you need some padding for your head, use a thinly folded blanket or yoga mat (cushions are too unstable). A carpeted floor is ideal.

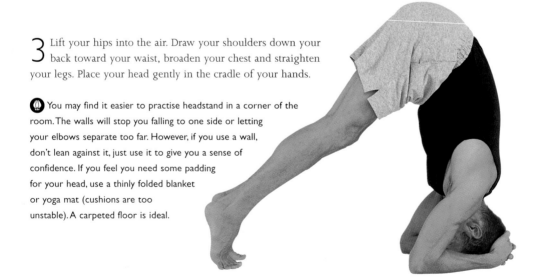

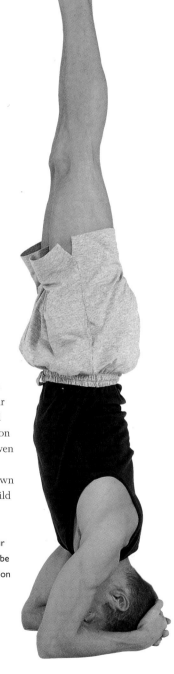

4 Your forearms now take most of your body weight and your neck should feel long, loose and free. Walk your feet toward your head as far as you can, engage your abdominal muscles, bend your legs and softly lift your knees toward your chest. Balance. Try to keep your shoulders moving in the direction of your waist. Lift your hips and keep your knees bent. Breathe steadily.

Once you have mastered the headstand you can try an alternative way of getting into the posture. When you are in step three, place your head on the floor and walk your feet toward your head. Instead of bending your legs, keep them straight as you lift them off the ground and move them slowly upward to point to the ceiling. You need considerable abdominal strength to enter headstand in this way, and you will need to draw up your abdominal muscles strongly.

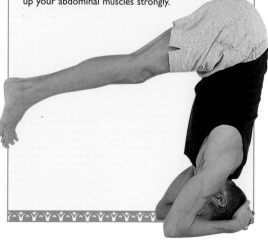

5 When your hips and torso are aligned, straighten your legs. Flex your feet slightly and imagine that you are standing on the ceiling. Keep your breath even and regular. Stay as long as is comfortable and then come down gently, with control. Rest in child pose (see page 68).

Being upside-down changes our perspective on the world. This can be a settling experience in which tension is allowed to flow away. Try to imagine the body as a lightning conductor earthing all the mind's fizzing energy.

# plough and shoulderstand

HALASANA and SARVANGASANA  Plough and shoulderstand are wonderful upper back, and neck stretches with many of the benefits of inversion, such as resting the heart and improving circulation and the blood supply to the brain. The poses can help to relieve bloating, tension and insomnia. They promote relaxation and give you renewed energy and powers of concentration. Both poses stimulate the thyroid and parathyroid glands in the neck, which control the body's metabolism.

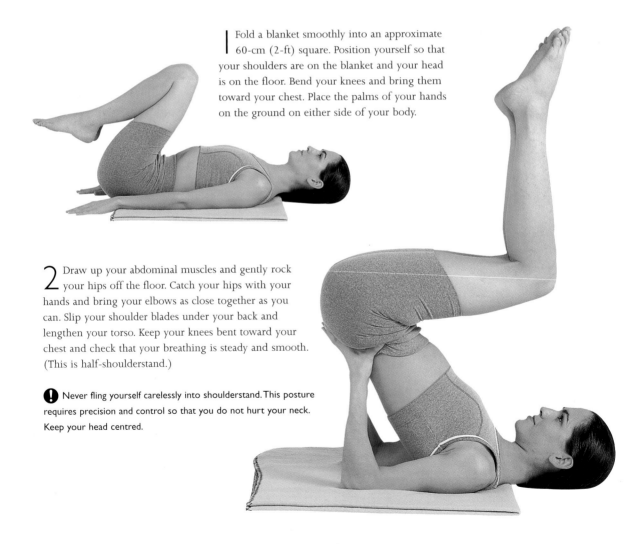

1 Fold a blanket smoothly into an approximate 60-cm (2-ft) square. Position yourself so that your shoulders are on the blanket and your head is on the floor. Bend your knees and bring them toward your chest. Place the palms of your hands on the ground on either side of your body.

2 Draw up your abdominal muscles and gently rock your hips off the floor. Catch your hips with your hands and bring your elbows as close together as you can. Slip your shoulder blades under your back and lengthen your torso. Keep your knees bent toward your chest and check that your breathing is steady and smooth. (This is half-shoulderstand.)

⚠ Never fling yourself carelessly into shoulderstand. This posture requires precision and control so that you do not hurt your neck. Keep your head centred.

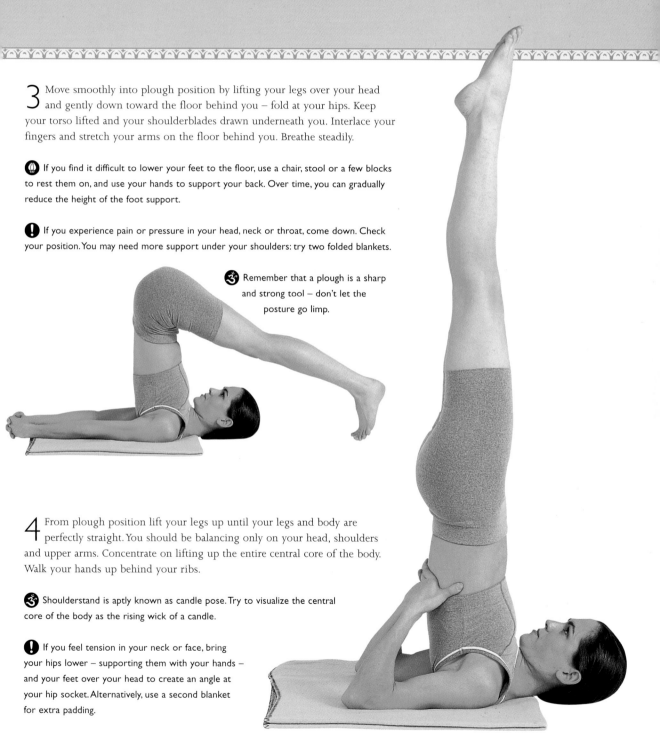

3 Move smoothly into plough position by lifting your legs over your head and gently down toward the floor behind you – fold at your hips. Keep your torso lifted and your shoulderblades drawn underneath you. Interlace your fingers and stretch your arms on the floor behind you. Breathe steadily.

🌸 If you find it difficult to lower your feet to the floor, use a chair, stool or a few blocks to rest them on, and use your hands to support your back. Over time, you can gradually reduce the height of the foot support.

❗ If you experience pain or pressure in your head, neck or throat, come down. Check your position. You may need more support under your shoulders: try two folded blankets.

🕉 Remember that a plough is a sharp and strong tool – don't let the posture go limp.

4 From plough position lift your legs up until your legs and body are perfectly straight. You should be balancing only on your head, shoulders and upper arms. Concentrate on lifting up the entire central core of the body. Walk your hands up behind your ribs.

🕉 Shoulderstand is aptly known as candle pose. Try to visualize the central core of the body as the rising wick of a candle.

❗ If you feel tension in your neck or face, bring your hips lower – supporting them with your hands – and your feet over your head to create an angle at your hip socket. Alternatively, use a second blanket for extra padding.

# fish

MATSYASANA  Matsya is an incarnation of the Indian god Vishnu, who turned himself into a fish to save the world from a flood. Fish has a strong effect on *anahata* and *vishudda chakras* (see page 25). It bends the upper body gracefully backward and strengthens the spine, neck, chest and respiratory system. Fish is an ideal counterpose to shoulderstand (see pages 86–7). Avoid fish if it causes dizziness or nausea.

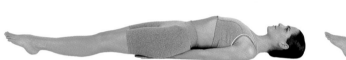

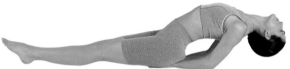

1 Lying down, bring your hands underneath you, palms face-down and elbows straight. Draw your shoulder blades together and down. Lift your chest slightly. Stretch your legs. Keep your ankles, thighs and knees together.

2 Breathe in and bend your arms as you raise your chest and head. Rotate your shoulder blades back and down. Lift your abdominals, keep your legs strong and your chest broad. Direct your breath into the top four ribs.

3 Delicately lower the crown of your head until it just touches the floor – there should be very little weight on it and you should not feel any compression of the head or neck. Keep your chest lifted and stay in this position for a few breaths.

🕉 In this pose, try to cultivate a feeling of floating.

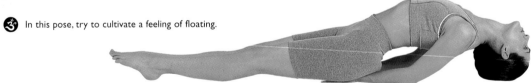

🪷 If you can hold fish with ease, remove your hands from under your body and stretch your arms up toward the ceiling and bring your palms together. Alternatively, take your hands over your head to touch the floor behind you. Don't lose the height in your chest or the lightness of your head – try to dive into the pose as if you were swimming. Breathe. Replace your arms, then slowly lower your head and chest. Relax.

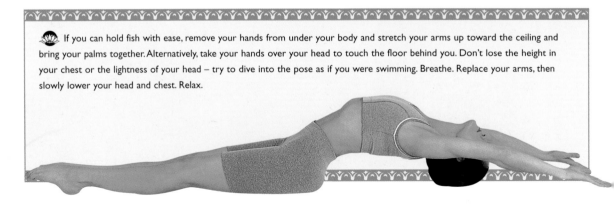

# corpse pose

SAVASANA  Doing the corpse pose at the end of your *asana* practice allows all your body systems to relax and to assimilate the work that you have done. It is also highly effective in other ways; for example, it can be used at the beginning of your practice session to prepare your mind for *asana*, and on its own to calm and centre your mind and body when you are feeling tense and when you are tired and need a quick way of reinvigorating yourself.

🕉 It is important that you feel relaxed and comfortable in this pose as the aim is to release any tension from your mind and body. Make sure that you are warm enough – many people like to put on extra clothes and a pair of socks, or cover themselves with a blanket, for this stage of their yoga practice (the body cools down during relaxation).

❗ If you are more than five months pregnant, it is not advisable to lie on your back for very long. Instead, lie on your left side with a cushion under your knee and a block or pillow under your head to support your neck.

🔥 If your low back or neck is stiff or sore, put a block under your head. Bend your knees; feet flat on the floor 45 cm (18 in) apart. Bring your knees together.

Lie on your back with your feet slightly apart. Relax your ankles and knees, and your buttock muscles. Move your arms a little way from your torso, turn the palms of your hands upward and relax your arms. Move your shoulders away from your head – make them broad. Relax your head, neck and face. Let your face be level – your chin should be neither sticking up nor pressed down. Close your eyes and let your breath become soft and subtle and your mind become still. If your mind wanders, gently bring your attention back to your breathing. Allow your body to soften and sink into the ground. Direct your breath into any areas of tension and allow them melt to away. Rest like this for 10 minutes, or longer if you wish. To come out of the pose, stretch your arms over your head, then bend your knees and roll to your right side. Slowly come up to a sitting position.

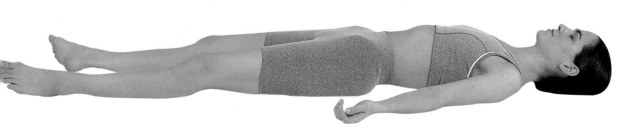

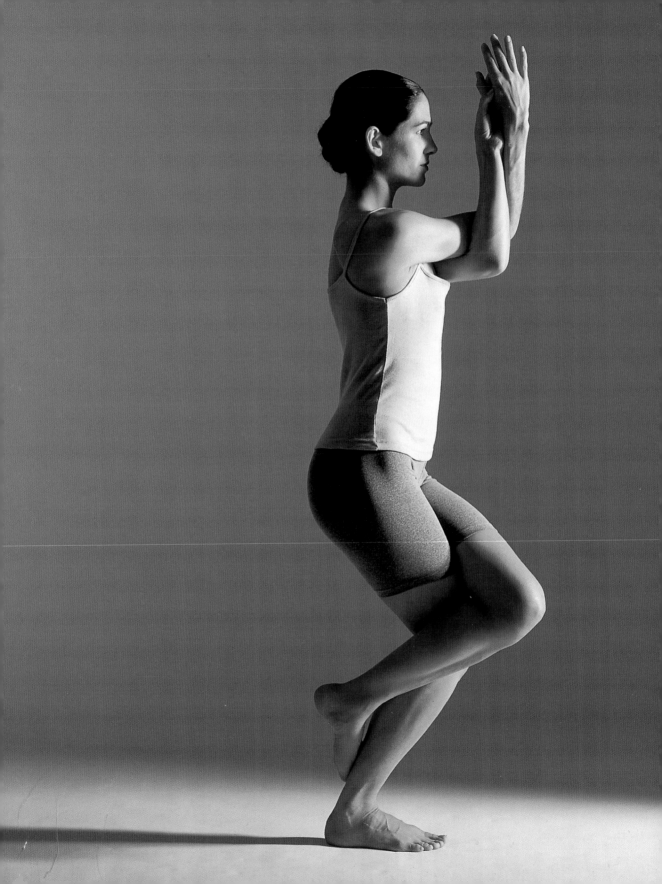

# sequences of *asanas*

A varied posture practice keeps your
understanding of yoga alive and growin
By doing a sequence of postures, you
systematically through all muscle gro
energy and allowing it to circulate sm
around your body.

This chapter includes the well-known sun
salutation sequence, suggestions for strong
and softer sequences and ways of closing your
practice. All the sequences are based upon the
poses given in Chapter 4. You can adapt each
sequence to suit your time, energy levels and
ability or you can create your own sequence.
Allow each posture to flow into the next in the
way that feels most natural to you – trust your
intuition to guide you from pose to pose.
Remember to perform asymmetrical postures
on both sides of your body. Finally, try not to
avoid postures that you find difficult – do an easier
modification or an alternative variation if you need
to, but do the posture.

# energizing morning sequence

The following series of postures can provide a dynamic start to the day – try to set aside some time in your morning routine to practise. If you can, face the sun as you practise – think of the sequence as a revital[...]g way to greet the day. We all naturally feel stiffer in the morning than the evening, so don't h[...]d if th[...] first few postures in your morning sequence feel a little tight. Breathe into each pose [...] your body loosening up as you move into it. Take your time and allow yourself a relaxing

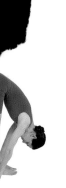

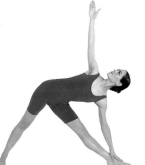

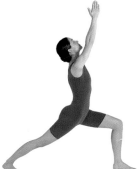

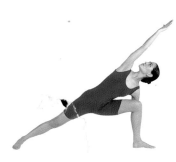

**1: STANDING FORWARD BEND**
(page 55)

**2: TRIANGLE**
(page 56)

**3: WARRIOR POSE**
(page 60)

**4: EXTENDED-ANGLE POSE**
(page 59)

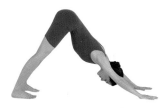

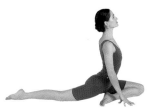

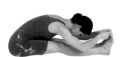

**5: DOWN-FACING DOG**
(page 62)

**6: PIGEON POSE**
(page 80)

**7: CAMEL POSE**
(page 69)

**8: SITTING FORWARD BEND**
(page 72)

posture at intervals if you need it. Build up to the full sequence over time. Remember to practise any asymmetrical postures on both sides of your body. You could extend the practice by beginning with a few rounds of full- or half-sun salutation (see pages 100–102). Make sure that you leave plenty of time for the final relaxation posture – it is crucial for clearing the mind, as well as letting the changes that have taken place during the sequence filter through the body.

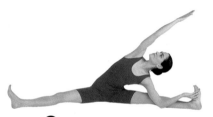

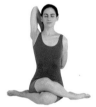

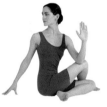

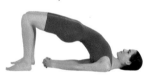

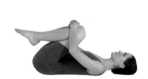

9: SITTING LEG STRETCH
(page 71)

10: COW-FACE POSE
(page 70)

11: TWIST B
(page 78)

12: BRIDGE POSE
(page 77)

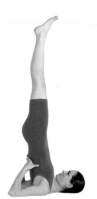

13: SHOULDERSTAND
(pages 86–7)

14: KNEES-TO-CHEST POSE
(page 76)

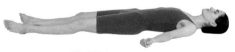

15: CORPSE POSE
(page 89)

# evening sequence

This sequence is an excellent way to unwind after a long, tiring day, and to free stress and aid digestion and sleep. The postures help to open and extend both the front and back surfaces of the body, relieving feelings of tension, particularly around the upper back, neck and shoulders – ideal if you work in a sedentary job and spend most of your day sitting at a desk. Prepare with a few rounds of full- or half-sun salutation (see pages 100–102). Evening sequence should be performed as smoothly and fluidly

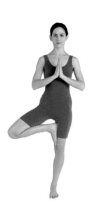

I: TREE POSE
(page 64)

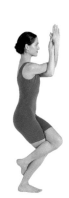

2: EAGLE POSE
(page 65)

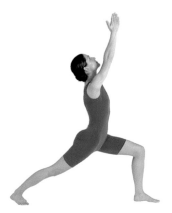

3: WARRIOR POSE
(page 60)

4: DOWN-FACING DOG
(page 62)

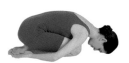

5: CHILD POSE
(page 68)

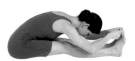

6: SITTING FORWARD BEND
(page 72)

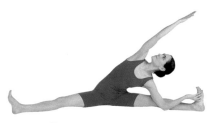

7: SITTING LEG STRETCH
(page 71)

as possible – listen to your intuition and allow it to guide you freely in to and out of each posture (as always, remember to do asymmetrical postures on both sides of your body). Try to stay in each pose for at least two to five breaths. Taking care to breathe evenly and steadily, allow energy to radiate through the body with each breath. Imagine the tension in your legs draining out through your feet, and the tightness in your neck and shoulders evaporating from your head.

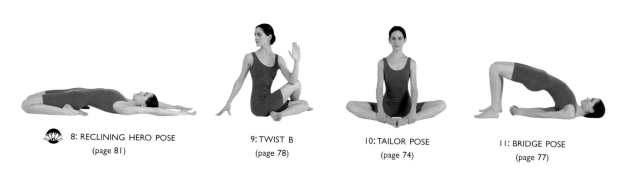

8: RECLINING HERO POSE
(page 81)

9: TWIST B
(page 78)

10: TAILOR POSE
(page 74)

11: BRIDGE POSE
(page 77)

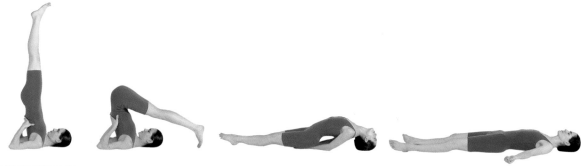

12: SHOULDERSTAND
(pages 86–7)

13: PLOUGH
(pages 86–87)

14: FISH
(page 88)

15: CORPSE POSE
(page 89)

# gentle sequence

This sequence is the perfect way to start building your posture practice if you are relatively new to yoga or wish to start practising again after a long break. The sequence's calming effect makes it great to do after a stressful day, no matter what your ability. The series contains a range of forward-, backward- and side-bending postures with balances and twists. Opt for an easier variation (particularly with step 7, cobra; step 9, sitting forward bend; and step 11, cow-face pose) if you need to. Remember, the postures

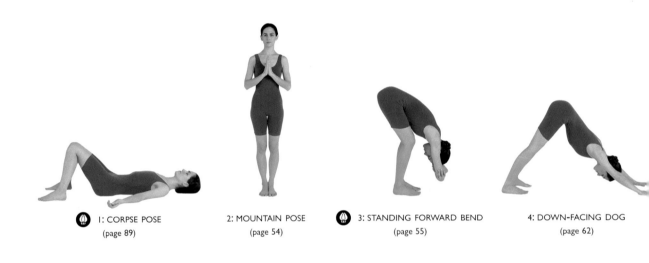

1: CORPSE POSE
(page 89)

2: MOUNTAIN POSE
(page 54)

3: STANDING FORWARD BEND
(page 55)

4: DOWN-FACING DOG
(page 62)

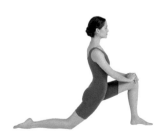
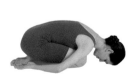
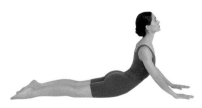
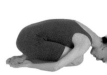

5: CRESCENT-MOON POSE
(pages 66–7)

6: CHILD POSE
(page 68)

7: COBRA
(page 73)

8: CHILD POSE
(page 68)

should be steady and comfortable – it is much better to do an easier variation than to struggle with the full posture. Complete the sequence once, staying in each posture for two or three breaths, gradually working up to more breaths over time. Asymmetrical poses should be worked through on both sides. Develop awareness of your breathing and of the way in which gravity acts on the body. The sequence will enhance spinal flexibility, tone your digestive system, and will generally improve mobility.

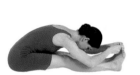

9: SITTING FORWARD BEND
(page 72)

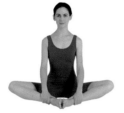

10: TAILOR POSE
(page 74)

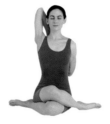

11: COW-FACE POSE
(page 70)

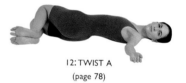

12: TWIST A
(page 78)

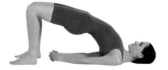

13: BRIDGE POSE
(page 77)

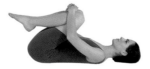

14: KNEES-TO-CHEST POSE
(page 76)

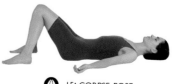

15: CORPSE POSE
(page 89)

# strong sequence

This sequence of postures will help you to develop stamina, flexibility and balance. You need to have a thorough knowledge of the individual poses before you attempt them in series. Warm up with several rounds of sun salutation (see pages 100–101), and then work through the following postures carefully (always doing asymmetrical poses on both sides of the body). Hold each posture for at least five breaths. As you become familiar with the sequence, focus your attention on how each posture works on your

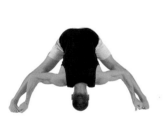

1: HANDS-TO-FEET POSE
(page 58)

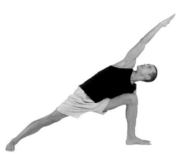

2: EXTENDED-ANGLE POSE
(page 59)

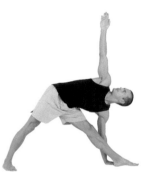

3: TRIANGLE
(page 56)

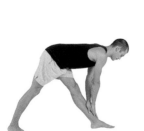

4: REVOLVED SIDE STRETCH
(page 57)

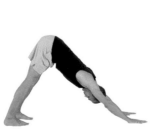

5: DOWN-FACING DOG
(page 62)

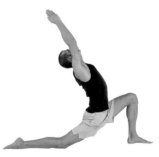

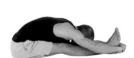 6: CRESCENT-MOON POSE
(pages 66–7)

7: SITTING FORWARD BEND
(page 72)

body, mind and emotions. Try focusing on the integration of your breathing with the movements: how does this feel? Can you develop the posture by breathing more fully? Are you holding your breath as the effort increases? You can also vary the practice by focusing on a specific part of your body, such as your hands or feet. If your hands are joined, imagine *prana* looping continuously around your body. If your feet are planted firmly on the floor, find a way to let them "root" into the earth. Keep experimenting!

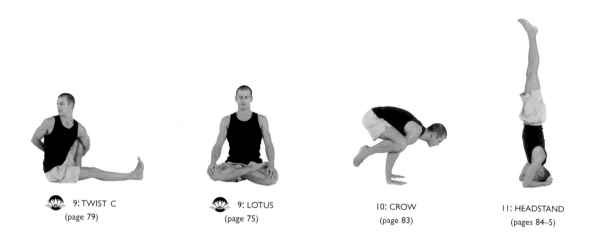

9: TWIST C
(page 79)

9: LOTUS
(page 75)

10: CROW
(page 83)

11: HEADSTAND
(pages 84–5)

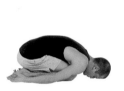
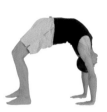
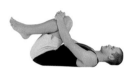
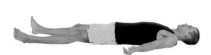

12: CHILD POSE
(page 68)

13: WHEEL
(page 82)

14: KNEES-TO-CHEST POSE
(page 76)

15: CORPSE POSE
(page 89)

# sun salutation

This sequence of postures has been practised for hundreds of years, traditionally facing the rising sun. The salutation makes a stimulating warm-up for any posture practice at any time of day – the rhythmic breathing and the deep, expansive movements generate considerable body heat, aiding flexibility. The sequence consists of forward- and backward-bending postures which, linked together in a continuous

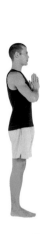

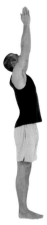

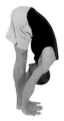

1: stand, feet together and hands at centre of chest

2: lift your arms overhead

3: fold forward

4: drop your left leg back into a deep lunge

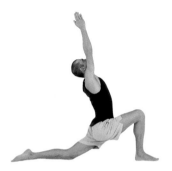

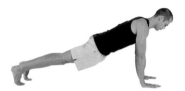

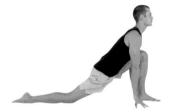

5: raise your arms overhead and look up

6: drop your hands to the floor; step back to a flat-back position

7: lower your knees, chest and forehead to the floor

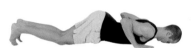

flow, help to develop strength and an awareness of your breathing. Try to perform the sequence at least six times, allowing one repetition to flow into the next (lead alternately with each leg). If you don't have much time, the sun salutation makes the ultimate, complete short yoga practice. Try the half-sun salutation on the following page if you are stiff, injured or a beginner.

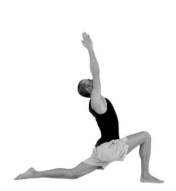

8: push gently forward into cobra (page 73)

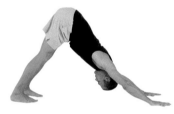

9: press your hips back and up into down-facing dog (page 62)

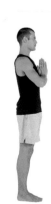

10: step forward with your right foot

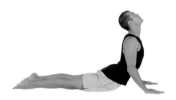

11: lift your arms overhead and look up

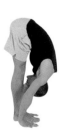

12: drop your hands to the floor, step your feet together, fold into forward bend

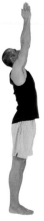

13: lift your arms overhead

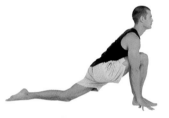

14: return to starting position

## ☸ HALF-SUN SALUTATION

This sequence is a gentle version of sun salutation (see pages 100–101) and is an ideal warm-up for an *asana* practice if you are new to yoga, you feel stiff or tired or you simply want a gentle practice. Focus on co-ordinating your breath with your movements. Take an in-breath each time you lift your body and an out-breath each time you fold forward. You can repeat this sequence as many times as you like; try to do four to six rounds for maximum benefit and reinvigoration.

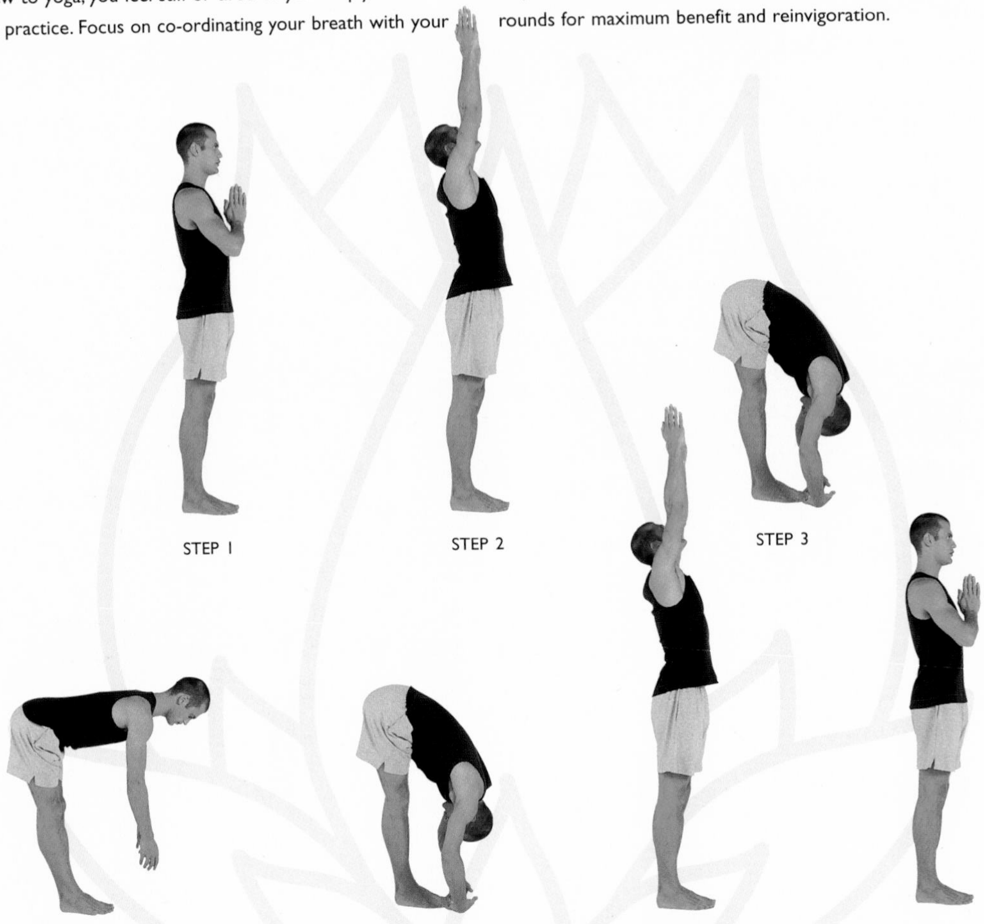

STEP 1

STEP 2

STEP 3

STEP 4

STEP 5

STEP 6

STEP 7

# closing your practice

Either of these short sequences can be used to close an *asana* practice. They each extend and relax your spine in preparation for corpse pose (see page 89). Choose the strong sequence to close a dynamic *asana* practice when you are feeling energetic. The soft sequence consists of moderate spinal stretches and is a good ending to a gentle practice or if you are feeling tired.

 STRONG

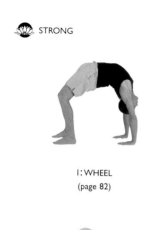

I: WHEEL
(page 82)

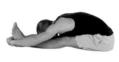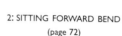

2: SITTING FORWARD BEND
(page 72)

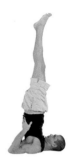

3: SHOULDERSTAND
(pages 86–7)

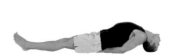

4: PLOUGH
(pages 86–7)

5: FISH
(page 88)

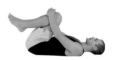

6: KNEES-TO-CHEST POSE
(page 76)

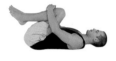 SOFT

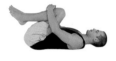

I: KNEES-TO-CHEST POSE
(page 76)

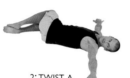

2: TWIST A
(page 78)

3: HALF-SHOULDERSTAND
(page 86)

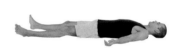

4: CORPSE POSE
(page 89)

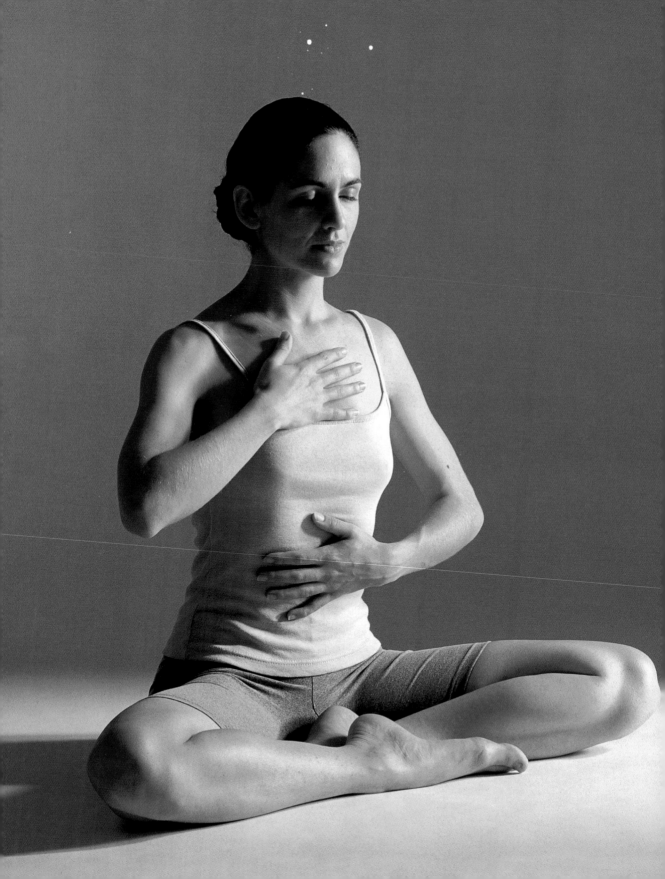

# the vital breath

The gentle rhythm of our breathing is our constant companion from the day we are born until the day we die. By learning to first observe and then to control our breathing, we can influence our emotional state, our ability to concentrate and the way energy moves in our bodies. *Pranayama* ("breath control") exercises form a practical link between the mind, the physical body and the subtle body (see page 21), and are a fundamental part of yoga practice.

In this chapter we look at the importance of breathing in yoga, as well as specific exercises that focus on the subtle aspect of breath and the movement of *prana*.

# *pranayama*: breath control

According to the *Upanishads* (see page 17), breath control is an essential part of yoga practice
– only by extending the breath can the yogi learn to tame and channel *prana* and reach higher states
of consciousness. The text of the *Upanishads* compares a person who practices yoga without breath
control to someone setting sail across an ocean in an unbaked earthenware boat – the boat will soon
absorb water and sink!

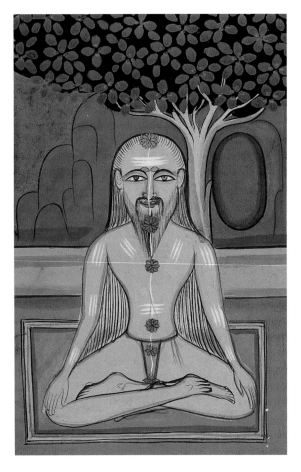

In this 18th-century manuscript painting, the yogi is seen in the lotus
position (see page 75), which balances the body perfectly and is an ideal
posture for pranayama practice.

Compared with all our other body systems, our respiratory system is unique. On the one hand it is involuntary (we continue to breathe even when we are unconscious), while on the other hand it is voluntary in that we can control it by deliberately lengthening, shortening or holding our breath. In Hatha yoga we learn to control the breath extremely accurately using a range of techniques known collectively as *pranayama*. In this way, our breath becomes a tool which can be used to regulate our physical and emotional states, and which eventually can lead us to a state of bliss or enlightenment. The text of the *Hathayoga Pradipika* (see pages 16–17) explains that when the breath is steady, so is the mind.

Yogis who devote hours of every day to *pranayama* practice can perform extraordinary feats of breath control, including slowing down the breath and the heart rate until they are virtually undetectable. However, far more important than any physical skill, is the practitioners' ability to free themselves from the obstructions of negative thoughts or a wandering mind. Because *pranayama* facilitates mental focus it is an essential preparation for and aid to the practice of meditation.

According to the 17th-century text *Gheranda Samhita* (see page 17), there are four requisites for *pranayama* practice. The first is *sthana* ("right place") – somewhere cool, quiet and, ideally, away from any distractions. The second is *kala* ("right time") – choose a time when you will be undisturbed; if possible, practice before dawn (although any time is better than not at all). The third is *mita-ahara* ("right diet"), you should be neither hungry nor too full, having eaten in moderation. The fourth is *nadi-suddhi* which refers to the purity of the energy channels (*nadis*) through which *prana* flows (see pages 20–23). These principles still apply today as they did 400 years ago.

## Extending the breath

According to one yogic tradition, we are born with a certain number of breaths for a lifetime. Yogis who watched the breathing rates of animals, noticed that those with slow rates of breathing, such as elephants and pythons, lived longer than faster-breathing species. By slowing down our breathing – extending each breath to gain from it the maximum benefit to our body, mind and spirit – we are able to prolong our life. Although in a literal sense this may seem farfetched, slowing down our breathing reduces our stress levels enabling us to relax and enjoy each moment of life more fully. Slowing down the breath also has a beneficial effect on the heart, which may help to prolong life.

## Inhalation, breath retention and exhalation

*Pranayama* is divided into three phases: inhalation (*puraka*), breath retention (*kumbhaka*; when the breath is held in the lungs), and exhalation (*rechaka*). The inhalation is a nourishing breath that brings energy, warmth, strength and vitality to the mind and body. Retaining, or holding, the breath creates a clear pathway around our body that allows *prana* to move freely into all areas, filling us with energy. The exhalation is cleansing, cooling, restorative, calming and balancing. A single, complete breath, taken fully, is both nourishing and energizing. Some *pranayama* exercises are based on manipulating the duration of *puraka*, *kumbhaka* and *rechaka*.

## Starting *pranayama*

Yoga texts recommend that beginners undertake *pranayama* for between five and ten minutes at a time. Accomplished yogis can practice for up to an hour. Just as the muscles

### BANDHAS: THE LOCKS OF YOGA

The *bandhas* are "locks" – muscular movements that seal *prana* into certain areas of the body or re-direct its flow elsewhere in the body. They can be practised on their own or combined with *asana*, *pranayama* or *mudra* (see page 119). Muscles can be contracted strongly or gently.

There are three *bandhas*. *Jalandhara bandha*, at the throat, is performed by lifting the chest and bringing the chin downward and inward while holding the breath. *Uddiyana* ("upward flying") *bandha* consists of lifting the abdominal muscles upward and inward after exhaling completely, and can also refer to a contraction of the lowest part of the abdomen, below the navel. In *astanga vinyasa* yoga, *uddiyana bandha* can be held with *mula bandha* during *asana*. *Mula* ("root") *bandha* consists of lifting the pelvic floor muscles to contract the perineum upward into the body. When all three locks are performed together, they form *maha bandha*, the great seal.

Although the specific practice of *bandha* is beyond the scope of this book, you may be able to observe the effects of holding or releasing *mula bandha* and *uddiyana bandha* during posture practice (contract only the lower part of the abdomen when you do *uddiyana bandha*).

that control our limbs become stiff through everyday misuse or lack of use, so do the muscles involved in our breathing. We would not, for example, expect to be able to achieve the lotus position without a considerable amount of practice, so we should not expect to undertake *pranayama* without similar preparation. If you feel tired, dizzy or "strange" when you practise, you are doing too much too fast – take it slowly. Make sure you avoid straining when you practise *pranayama* – air should pour into your lungs easily and this should always feel comfortable.

# the effects of *pranayama*

The basic function of breathing is to bring life-force – *prana* – into the body. In addition, *pranayama* allows us to develop more control over our breathing (the word *ayama* means "control", "direction" or "expansion"), so that we can use our breath in a variety of beneficial ways. For example, different breathing techniques can energize the body, clear the mind, reduce physical pain, improve concentration, alleviate anxiety or induce a state of relaxation.

Most people do not breathe in a way that fully utilizes all the space in their lungs. We are rarely encouraged to think about our breathing and the effect that it has on our mental and physical states. The first step in *pranayama* is the non-judgmental observation of your natural breathing. If you try the exercise on page 111 (observing the breath)

you may be surprised in two ways: first, the pattern of your breath may be erratic (short breaths, long breaths, with uneven gaps between them); second, you may find that it is difficult to concentrate on your breathing, even for a few seconds without becoming distracted. (You can help the mind to focus on the breath by repeating silently: "I am aware I am breathing in, I am aware I am breathing out" as you focus on the breath.)

Once you have gained a basic awareness of your breath, you can learn specific *pranayama* exercises (see pages 110–13) that will help you to develop a great deal of control over your body and your emotional and mental states. In yoga classes, students usually learn *pranayama* in conjunction with or after *asana*. As the *Hathayoga Pradipika* (see pages 16–17) says: once we are "established in *asana* and having control of the body, taking a balanced diet; *pranayamas* should be practised".

## Physical benefits of *pranayama*

*Pranayama* is recognized as a means of rejuvenating the body, and it is known to have enormous curative value – by increasing the intake of oxygen into the body, it fully replenishes the blood supply with oxygen so that all our internal organs gain the nourishment they need. In turn, this enables our body systems, such as the digestive system, to work more effectively. Increased oxygen intake is particularly beneficial for the functioning of the kidneys, liver and spleen. The texts of yoga recommend *pranayama* as an effective cure for a range of ailments from

### TIPS FOR *PRANAYAMA* PRACTICE

- If you intend to practise *pranayama* after *asana*, relax between the two (see page 89); alternatively, practise *pranayama* first.
- Sit upright in a comfortable position for *kapalabhati*, *anuloma viloma*, *sithali* and *sitkari* (see pages 110–113). Any of the suggested meditation postures on pages 118–119 are appropriate.
- Sit, or lie down in corpse pose (see page 89), for *ujjayi*, *brahmari* and extended breath exercises (see pages 110–113).
- Always breathe through your nose (except during *sithali* and *sitkari*; see page 113).
- In yoga, the out-breath is calming and balancing. Generally make your out-breaths the same length or longer than your in-breaths.
- The best preparation for *pranayama* is *asana*, so if you are finding *pranayama* difficult, go back to *asana* practice and observe your breath as you perform the postures.

hiccoughs to headache and earache, as well as serious complaints such as asthma. The stress-relieving effects of *pranayama* can help prevent a wide range of stress-related symptoms and illnesses.

Pranayama practice strengthens all of the muscles involved in breathing and helps to expand the capacity of the lungs. Meanwhile, you can use your breath to relieve tension in other parts of your body. The simplest way to do this is to direct your in-breath to a particular part of your body – your lower back, for example. By breathing out "from" this area you can let the point of tension soften and be carried away with your breath.

## Emotional benefits of *pranayama*

Mood and emotions are closely linked with breathing patterns. To understand how they are connected think about how your breathing changes when you feel excited or nervous. States of agitation generally cause the breath to become quick, shallow and uneven (this can create a negative loop in which our breathing exacerbates the original anxiety). In contrast, when we feel relaxed we are more likely to breathe slowly and evenly. In *pranayama*, we develop the ability to calm and control the breath – and in this way we are able to focus the mind and manage the emotions.

## *PRANAYAMA* AND THE RESPIRATORY SYSTEM

The respiratory system relies upon the effective use of several muscles. The largest of these is the diaphragm, the sheet of muscle lying under the lungs, which is attached to the spine and lower rib cage. As we inhale, the diaphragm moves down toward the abdominal area. This lowers the atmospheric pressure in the chest and air rushes into the lungs to equalize the pressure. The rib cage lifts and opens to create space. As we breathe out, the diaphragm relaxes back into its arched position, and the ribs move down and air is pushed out. When we shallow-breathe, the diaphragm is not fully utilized. We use only part of our lungs' capacity, and retain stale breath as we breathe out. Through *pranayama* we breathe using the diaphragm fully; the upper and lower lungs are completely filled with air and stale breathe is fully exhaled.

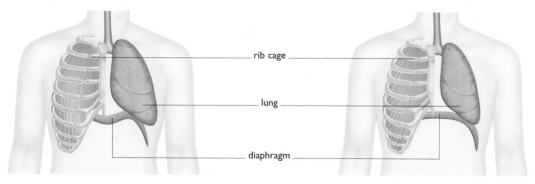

rib cage

lung

diaphragm

INHALATION

EXHALATION

# *pranayama* exercises

The following exercises explain how to regulate your breath in a variety of ways. Techniques include controlling the movement of your diaphragm, changing the pressure and sound of your breath as it moves through your throat and manipulating the lengths of your in-breath and out-breath. Each exercise has a specific effect – some are energizing, and others are tranquilizing – but all will enhance the flow of *prana*.

Before you try any of the following *pranayama* exercises you should feel comfortable practising the concentration exercise described in the box on the page opposite.

## *Kapalabhati*: the shining skull

Literally translated, the Sanskrit name for this exercise means "skull shining" and this is a bit what it feels like. *Kapalabhati* is an exercise in diaphragmatic control and uses a "pumping" breath action that produces mental clarity and perspective. If you feel sluggish and lethargic, it can help to restore energy. In physical terms, the exercise strengthens the diaphragm, and tones the heart, liver and stomach. *Kapalabhati* is also a *kriya* (cleansing exercise) for the respiratory system and the *nadis* (see page 23). It clears out blockages, allowing energy and oxygen to flow freely. You should avoid practising this exercise if you are pregnant or suffer from high blood pressure, depression, panic attacks, anxiety, epilepsy or diabetes.

*Kapalabhati*, like most other breathing exercises, should be practised in rounds. Start by taking a couple of normal breaths. Then inhale through your nose. Now contract your abdominal muscles sharply to exhale forcefully through your nose. (Your exhalation should be similar to the action of blowing out a candle, but using your nose rather than your mouth.) As your diaphragm releases you will automatically inhale gently. Repeat the pumping action of the exhalation together with the passive in-breaths in four short, rhythmic bursts. Then take a deep in-breath and exhale normally. This is one complete round of *kapalabhati* and you should repeat it four times. Gradually build up to four rounds of 20 breaths.

## Ujjayi: the victorious breath

This is a simple breathing exercise, which can be used alone or in combination with other breathing exercises. You can also try it during posture practice. The technique consists of making a gentle, continuous hissing sound on both the in- and the out-breath by contracting your throat muscles slightly. The sound gives the mind something to focus upon. (It sounds similar to putting a shell to your ear to listen to the "sea".) As you control the pressure of the breath it becomes very slow and even. Ujjayi has a tranquilizing effect and renews energy and concentration. The exercise tones the respiratory system and internal organs and increases body heat.

To practise making the sound, breathe out through your mouth making a soft "haaa" noise as if steaming up a window. Now make the same noise with your mouth softly closed so that you are exhaling through your nose. Try to replicate the sound on your in-breath with your mouth still closed – you will need to use slightly different muscles in your throat. Repeat 12 breaths – and gradually increase – or use *ujjayi* in your *asana* practice. Ujjayi breathing does not have to be loud, just audible.

## Extending the breath and breath retention

This *pranayama* exercise involves holding your breath between inhaling and exhaling, and making your exhalation longer than your inhalation. It allows stale air to be expelled from the lungs, calms the nervous system and creates a feeling of tranquility. You may find it easier to practise this exercise while lying down. Once you are familiar with the technique, aim to practise sitting up.

Let your breathing settle and listen to it carefully. Monitor each breath to see if it is deep or shallow, slow or fast. Count how long each inhalation and exhalation takes. (You may find that you naturally count in time with your pulse rate – this, or any other rhythm is fine, as long as it is consistent.) Now, start to make your out-breaths longer until they are twice as long as your in-breaths – so

your in-breath might last for a count of 4 and your out-breath for a count of 8. Repeat this several times. Now focus your attention on the pause between each breath. Gently suspend or hold your breath at the top of each inhalation until you feel your out-breath rising – then exhale. This method of breathing is neither easy nor natural and it may take you some time to achieve. Aim eventually to hold your breath for three times longer than your in-breath. Use a 1:3:2 ratio in which, for example, you breathe in for a count of 4, hold your breath for a count of 12 and breathe out for a count of 8. As you finish breathing out, allow yourself a gentle, unforced pause

## OBSERVING THE BREATH

Before you attempt any of the other exercises in this chapter, work on this simple breath observation. You will be using a combination of concentration (*dharana*) and breathing work (*pranayama*).

Lie in corpse pose (see page 89) or sit cross legged, in half-lotus (see page 75) or in hero pose (see page 81; step 1). Make sure that your spine is straight. Close your eyes and, if you like, place your hands on your chest and upper abdomen to help you feel the movement of your breath. Listen to the flow of air into and out of your body. Visualize its path through your nostrils, down your throat, into your lungs, and from your lungs into your blood. As you breathe out, visualize this pathway in reverse. Notice how your in-breath feels cool at the upper part of your nostrils, and how your out-breath feels warm at the lower edge.

What is the texture of your breathing? Is it rough or smooth, fast or slow, even or uneven? Don't worry if your breath is rough, fast or uneven – the act of observation is the important thing and controlling the quality of your breath will come next. If your attention wanders, gently bring your focus back to the movement of each breath.

Observe your breath in this way for as long as you feel comfortable, then gradually allow your breathing to become smooth, slow and even. Your out-breath becomes the same length as your in-breath with brief, consistent pauses in between. It may help to count how long each in- and out-breath takes. Try to breathe steadily in this way for a few minutes. Extend the time you spend on this exercise until it becomes easy.

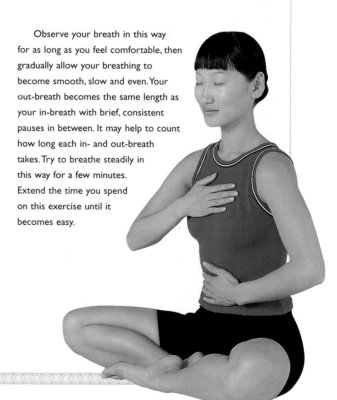

before breathing in again. As you become comfortable with this method of breathing, extend each stage of the breath, keeping to the same ratio; for example, breathe in for 6, hold for 18 and breathe out for 12. You can combine this exercise with ujjayi breathing (see page 110) if you wish.

### Anuloma viloma: alternate nostril breathing

You may not have noticed, but we breathe mostly through one nostril for an hour or so and then swap and breathe mostly through the other. In yoga this is explained by the fact that the two energy channels, ida and pingala, which exit at the nostrils, are constantly changing their dominance. Alternate nostril breathing balances the energies of ida and pingala.

Start by making the Vishnu mudra hand position: curl the index and middle fingers of your right hand into the palm. Now use your right thumb to close your right nostril. Inhale through your left nostril. Keeping your thumb

where it is, close the left nostril with your ring and little fingers and briefly hold your breath before releasing your thumb and exhaling through your right nostril. Now breathe in through your right nostril and close it again with your thumb. Hold your breath for a few moments, then release your fingers and exhale through the left nostril, keeping the right closed. These two breaths form one complete round. Repeat 12 rounds to begin with, increasing to 24 or more as your practice improves and you feel comfortable with the technique.

A variation of the alternate nostril breathing exercise involves placing your index and middle fingers on your forehead between your eyebrows, instead of curling them into your palm. This stimulates ajna chakra (see page 25) which is located at this point behind your forehead. By using this hand position you can charge ajna chakra with prana. This variation is a stronger practice than the basic alternate nostril breathing exercise and should be undertaken with care.

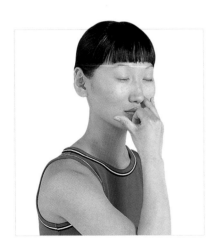

*This hand position, known as Vishnu mudra, is used during alternate nostril breathing. The middle and index fingers are curled into the palm of the hand and the thumb and remaining fingers are used alternately to close the right and left nostrils.*

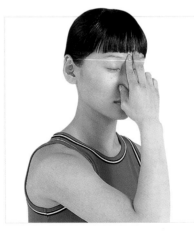

*This hand position can be used instead of vishnu mudra in alternate nostril breathing. The index and middle fingers rest on ajna chakra which is located between the eyebrows. This stimulates the flow of prana in ajna chakra.*

### Brahmari: humming-bee breath

This wonderfully-named prana-yama helps to focus your attention on your out-breath, enabling you to lengthen the out-breath while listening to its quality. Brahmari is said to make the voice sweet and is good for people, such as teachers, actors and singers, who rely heavily upon their voice. Brahmari can be profoundly relaxing, especially if you are suffering from tension in your neck, throat, upper back, or shoulders.

Start by inhaling fully through your nose. On your

## COUNTING THE ROUNDS

Keeping count of how many rounds of breathing you do in each exercise is a key part of pranayama. The mental focus required helps to improve your concentration in preparation for meditation – after all, if you are distracted you will lose count! The time-honoured way of counting the rounds is by using your own outstretched hand. Use your thumb to count along the finger-joints of the same hand in a spiral as shown. On the first round place your thumb on the base joint of your index finger; on the second, move up to the middle joint; on the third, up to the tip. Move across the tip joints of the other fingers for rounds 4 to 6; then, down the little finger for 7 and 8, across the base joints of the ring and middle fingers for 9 and 10 and up to and across the middle joints of the middle and ring fingers for 11 and 12.

The number of rounds you will do for each pranayama exercise varies, and suggestions are given in the individual instructions. As your practice develops, you will be able to increase the number of rounds that you do, but don't push yourself to do too much. Nine rounds of 12 breaths (108 repetitions) is known as a mala.

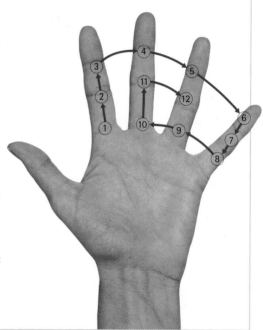

exhalation make a rounded and steady humming sound. Listen to the sound of the hum; vary its pitch, moving the sound around inside your head and chest. Eventually you will find a humming sound that feels comfortable. Make this sound on each inhalation and exhalation. Start with five to 10 breaths and build up gradually.

### Sithali: the cooling breath

This exercise has a cooling effect on the body and is fantastic if you are feeling hot and uncomfortable. Unusually for pranayama practice, the in-breath is taken through the mouth rather than the nose.

Roll your tongue and stick it out slightly, so that the tip just pokes out from your bottom lip. Inhale, drawing the air through the groove made by your curled tongue, as if sipping your breath in. Close your mouth and hold the breath for a few seconds. Exhale through your nose. Repeat the complete breath five to 10 times. (If you are unable to roll your tongue, practise the sitkari pranayama given below.)

### Sitkari: the sucking breath

This pranayama, like sithali, has an amazing cooling effect on the body, and also uses the mouth rather than the nose for the in-breath. Place the tip of your tongue on the roof of your mouth just behind your front teeth. On the in-breath draw the air in around the sides of your tongue – notice how cool it feels. Close your mouth and hold the breath for a few seconds before exhaling fully through your nose. Repeat the breath five to 10 times.

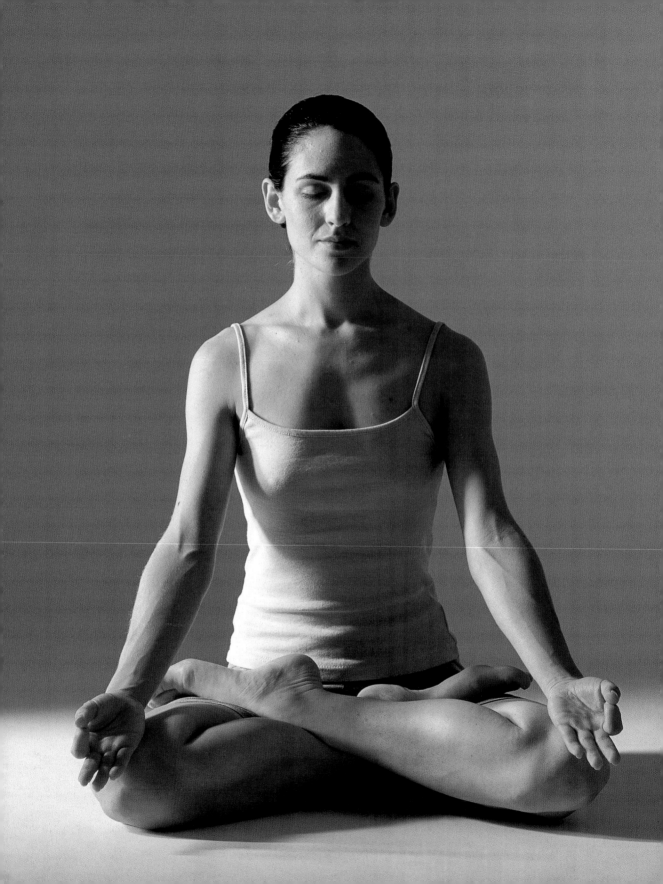

# meditation

Meditation is the active process of encouraging stillness in the mind. When practising meditation we temporarily withdraw the mind from the onslaught of daily pressures and tune into an inner oasis of calm. Even a few minutes of meditation each day can drastically improve our ability to cope with everyday life and help us to develop an awareness of our inner self.

Studies have shown that anxiety and stress levels can be reduced effectively through meditation, which also has a remarkable healing effect on the physical body. Requiring no athletic skill at all, meditation can be an ideal practice for those suffering illness or recovering from an injury.

This chapter discusses the discipline of meditation, including recommended sitting postures and the various tools, such as mantras, that we can use to help our practice.

# understanding meditation

People have been practising meditation – the act of completely stilling the mind into a state of total absorption or concentration – for centuries. We may experience something akin to meditation when we focus intensely on a game of a chess, a piece of music or a math problem. The difference between this state of mind and meditation is one of depth. Meditation is absolute – during meditation the mind and the subject of concentration become one. For many people, meditation marks the beginning of their spiritual path in yoga.

Meditation, or *dhyana*, is the seventh step in Patanjali's eight-fold path (see pages 18–19). His practical technique of focusing the mind takes us to the ultimate goal of yoga: *samadhi* – the attainment of self-realization and the state of becoming one with the universe or the "Absolute" (see page 14). On a more immediate level, meditation can be thought of as a way of quieting the buzz of images, thoughts and perceptions that crowd the mind during our waking lives.

Meditation involves a subtle act of "letting go" – and it is not something that you can learn through sheer hard work. Moving from ordinary consciousness into meditation is analogous to the transition between waking and sleeping – by nature it is not an action that can be willed. Also like sleep, meditation is not something that you are aware of when you are "in" it – you usually recognize a meditative state only after you have left it.

Practising *asana* provides a way of physically and mentally unwinding to help you to focus your mind in preparation for meditation. Some people benefit greatly from this kind of preparation, whereas others can slip into a meditative state comparatively easily without it. Don't worry about which group you fall into – it is the process of meditation that is important, not the route by which you get there. You may find that a moving meditation suits you best – some styles of yoga such as *astanga vinyasa* (see page 44) incorporate meditation into posture practice. The movement of the body provides a tool for concentrating the mind.

Apart from the spiritual goal of *samadhi*, there are many other benefits of meditation, such as stress relief, improved concentration, poise, equanimity and mental and emotional tranquility. Meditation can also help to heal physical ailments and reduce high blood pressure.

## Concrete and abstract meditation

Broadly speaking there are two types of meditation: concrete or *Saguna* (also known as qualified or formal meditation) and abstract or *Nirguna* (also known as "no mind", unqualified or formless meditation). The first type involves an external focus – usually an object, image, sound or symbol – which the yogi uses as a tool for concentration. This is generally assumed to be easier than abstract meditation because it gives the mind something solid, such as candle flame, to "attach" itself to. Abstract meditation has no external focus, and consists of absorption in the self (or the Absolute) – an abstract idea rather than an object. It is worth experimenting with both types – most people find that they are naturally drawn toward one or the other. Whichever you choose, both lead eventually to *samadhi*.

## Meditation practice

To begin meditation practice, find a quiet place where you will be warm, comfortable and undisturbed – the point of minimizing distractions is simply to make meditation easier. Try to make a habit of meditating in this place so that you learn to associate it with a state of focused concentration. If your meditation space is not as quiet or as private as you would like, just do the best with what you have. In theory, it is quite possible to meditate successfully in a street full of busy traffic!

Try not to practice meditation immediately after *asana* practice – either meditate beforehand or take a long period of rest and relaxation in the corpse pose before you begin meditation. Alternatively, practise *asana* and meditation at different times (unless of course you are practising *astanga vinyasa*).

Wear loose, comfortable clothing. Find a comfortable sitting position (see pages 118–9) and begin your chosen meditation exercise (see pages 120–3). If you lose concentration, gently and uncritically guide your mind back to the focus of the meditation, whether it is your breath, the flame of a candle, a mantra or a *yantra*. Don't rush at meditation – it comes in its own time – be patient and practice often.

Beginners should aim to meditate for 10 to 15 minutes at a time, if possible. Once you feel able to do this, try gradually to increase the length of each session until you are meditating for 30 minutes (longer if you wish) once or twice a day. However, if you find yourself sitting for 30 minutes fretting that you cannot focus your mind, you are probably trying to do too much too soon. As you become more experienced at meditation, you will gain a feel for how long you should practice.

*Whenever you have the opportunity, it can be wonderful to do your meditation practice outside in a beautiful and tranquil environment.*

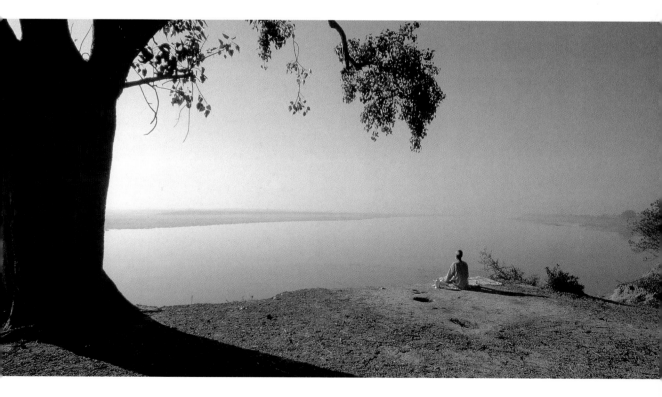

# meditation posture

How you sit when you meditate is crucial for the simple reason that if you are uncomfortable it will be difficult for you to concentrate. You must be able to stay in your chosen posture for a prolonged period without pain or discomfort. On the other hand, you shouldn't be so comfortable that you fall asleep! *Asana* practice can help you to develop the strength and flexibility that you need for some of the meditation postures, such as the full lotus.

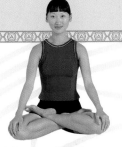

**FULL LOTUS**

One of the most important considerations when sitting down to meditate is the position of your spine, which should be long, upright and balanced to allow energy to flow freely and to ease the awakening of the higher energy centres in the body.

The traditional way to meditate is to sit on the floor. For some people, injuries in the low back, hips, hamstrings, knees or ankles make sitting on the floor uncomfortable. Many of us find it difficult simply because we spend prolonged periods of time sitting in chairs and our bodies have grown accustomed to this position. We need time – sometimes years – to train ourselves to sit comfortably on the floor again.

The following postures are suitable for meditation (you can also sit in a simple crossed-leg position). When you sit, use your hands to lift the fleshy part of your buttocks slightly up and out. This helps you to feel the sitting bones in firm contact with the floor (or chair) and minimizes the tendency to roll backward onto your sacrum.

### Sitting on a chair
If sitting on the floor for long periods is uncomfortable, begin by sitting in a chair. Choose a chair that is hard with a firm seat.

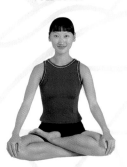

**HALF-LOTUS**

Avoid padded chairs or moulded plastic ones with scoop-shaped seats – they encourage the spine to collapse. Sit toward the front edge of your chair with your back lengthened and your feet flat on the floor, a little way apart (if your seat is too high, put some blocks or books under your feet). Rest your hands on your knees. You should feel balanced and at ease; you are aiming for a posture of minimal effort.

### Full lotus and half-lotus
The classic posture for meditation is full lotus (see page 75). Beginners to yoga often wonder why people bother to knot themselves up in this position. The reason is that in this posture the weight of the body becomes perfectly balanced. The legs and hips root down toward the earth and the spine rises effortlessly from this solid base. If you cannot do full lotus, try half-lotus, which also has a pleasantly grounding effect, but is a little more uneven. For this reason, alternate the lifted leg at each meditation session.

Even if you are not able to do them now, both lotus and half-lotus are worth working toward in your *asana* practice.

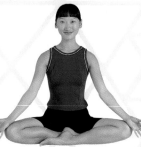

**HALF-ADEPTS POSE**

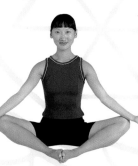

**TAILOR POSE**

## HAND POSITIONS FOR MEDITATION

The way you position your hands during meditation is a matter of personal choice – simply do whatever feels most comfortable. If you are sitting on a chair or in hero pose it may be easiest to place your hands on your thighs with your palms facing down. You can also use your hands to make various seals, known as *mudra* in Sanskrit. *Mudra* seal energy (*prana*; see pages 20–23) into the body or conduct its flow in a certain direction. As your sensitivity develops you may sense *prana* moving in different parts of your body. Performing *mudra* can be compared to completing an electrical circuit.

The classic *mudra* for meditation is known as the chin *mudra* or the "seal of consciousness". Hold your index finger and thumb together, with your palm upward. The nail of your index finger should touch the pad of your thumb. Chin *mudra* concentrates the flow of *prana* toward the higher *chakras* (see pages 24–27) in the body and aids concentration on the mind and the self.

## Half-adepts pose

This is a good alternative to the lotus variations – it puts considerably less strain on the knee joints, but provides a stable sitting position. Sit on the floor and cross your right foot in front of your body and bring your left foot in front of your right until your heels align. Alternate the forward foot at each meditation practice. Try to avoid tilting forward or letting your lower back collapse.

## Tailor pose

Tailor pose (see page 74) is another well-balanced posture. Try sitting on the edge of a folded blanket or block to elevate the hips slightly and counteract the tendency to roll backward. To alleviate pressure on the ankle bones, sit in the middle of a folded blanket. Sitting with your back against a wall is useful at first, but should not become a habit – leaning against anything throws the balance of the spine slightly off-centre making a posture hard to sustain.

## Hero pose

If you are uncomfortable in any of the previous postures, try sitting in hero pose (see page 81). This is an ideal intermediate stage between sitting in a chair and one of the crossed-leg poses. The full posture requires considerable knee, hip and ankle flexibility, but the following variation is suitable for most people. Kneel back on a pile of yoga blocks (or telephone directories) placed between your ankles. Use as many blocks as you need to feel comfortable. Whether you are sitting on one block or four, make sure that your sitting bones are perched just on the edge of them so that your thighs remain free. Keep your knees close together, your thigh bones parallel and the soles of your feet facing upward. Your head should now float weightlessly above your neck. Hero pose has a lovely sense of equilibrium about it – it is almost an effort to slouch!

If you have any discomfort in your ankles or the tops of your feet, place a rolled up mat or blanket just under your ankles and let your toes relax down toward the floor.

HERO POSE

# meditation techniques

The biggest challenge in meditation is training the mind to achieve and maintain a single point of focus. Many people find that a "tool", such as the breath, a mantra, a mandala or even something as simple as the flame of a candle, can help to concentrate the mind for successful meditation. At first you may find that you are simply concentrating on your chosen object, but with practice, concentration turns into contemplation and, eventually, you and your object become indistinguishable and you experience the goal of meditation – perfect, unified stillness.

The following techniques engage either your sense of hearing or your sense of sight. When you are first practising meditation, concentrating on a real sound or object can help you. When you are more experienced it may be sufficient to imagine the sound or object.

Try some or all of the following techniques to see which ones work best for you.

**Breath counting meditation**

This is a simple and traditional type of meditation that is different from the breathing exercises (*pranayama*) described on pages 110–113 in that here the breath is used as a focus for the mind. The sound of the breath forms its own natural mantra which is expressed as *So–Ham*: the in-breath is said to make the sound *So* and the out-breath *Ham*. This is translated as "I am He." In yogic terms, the word "He" refers to the universal spirit or the "Absolute". Breathing, therefore, is a constant, gentle reminder of the connection between the individual self and the universal consciousness.

To practise breath meditation sit comfortably in your chosen posture (see pages 118–19), close your eyes and listen to your breathing. Make no attempt to change its natural flow; just observe the breath as it is. Notice the point at which your breath touches the insides of your nostrils as you inhale and exhale. Let it become very

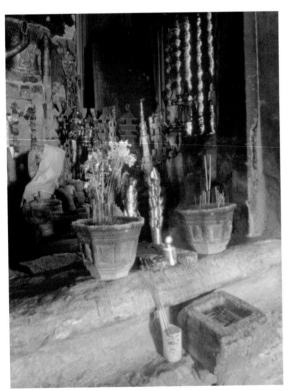

People all over the world use altars and sacred spaces as a focal point for prayer and meditation. When you start meditating you may find it useful to create a personal altar in your meditation space. This can be a small table or platform covered with a cloth. On this you can place a candle, fresh flowers, a statue, an OM symbol, a photograph or a picture of someone you respect such as a teacher, saint, god or holy person. These objects can set the mood for meditation and they can also be used as tools to concentrate the mind.

## OM MEDITATION

OM is the sacred sound of the universe; the single syllable to which the entire cosmos vibrates. It is a sacred mantra in the Hindu, Sikh, Jain and Buddhist traditions and symbolizes the universal spirit or the "Absolute" for yogis. The yogic text *Mandukya Upanishad* describes OM as follows: "OM symbolizes the supreme Reality, it is the past, present and future – everything is but the sound of OM."

Repeated aloud, the sound of OM is said to be the nearest that the human voice can come to the sound of the universal vibration. (It is thought by some that the mooing sound that cows make is also a representation of OM.)

There are four parts to the sound OM: "a", "u", "m" and the nasalized humming aftersound of the "m". (OM is spelled this way because the "a" and the "u" are merged together when OM is spoken.) These four parts relate to the different states of consciousness: waking, dreaming, deep dreamless sleep and the transcendental state. If you look at the Sanskrit symbol OM (shown left) you will see how these four parts are represented in its shape. The upper curve represents waking; the lower one dreaming; the wave-shape moving out from the centre, deep sleep; and the dot, the transcendental state. The crescent below the dot represents *maya* – illusion.

OM is sometimes referred to as the Mula-mantra (meaning "root mantra") and it is often used before and after another mantra (such as Gayatri-mantra; see main text, below).

Chanting OM to begin your meditation practice sets up an awareness of the vibration in your body, which you can follow with your mind. Let each repetition start at your navel and move up toward your forehead. Hold the humming M sound at the end the longest – you should be able to feel it vibrating in the bony parts of your skull. In the silence following the chanting of OM, try to feel the continued vibration in your body. Let your mind focus on this vibration and begin to listen for the inaudible sound of OM within your subtle body – silent meditation upon OM is thought to produce the truest sound.

subtle. Now begin to count your breaths from one to 10 and back again (each complete inhalation and exhalation counts as one). Use this simple counting routine as a way of keeping your mind focused. After a time you can stop counting and just listen to the steady rhythmic flow of your breath – it may become very slow during meditation. When your mind wanders, draw it back to the breath – resume counting if this helps you to concentrate.

### Mantra meditation

Mantras are repeated words that help to focus the mind during meditation. The word mantra means "thought expressed as sound". A mantra can be a single syllable, such as the holy syllable OM (see box, above), or a set of words, phrases or sounds. Some mantras are like prayers and have clear meanings. For example, a widely used Hindu yoga mantra – Gayatri-mantra – can be translated as: "OM, let us contemplate that celestial splendor of God Savitri so that he may inspire our visions." In contrast, the mantras that encapsulate the essence of each *chakra* (known as *bija* or seed mantras) are sounds with no literal meaning. For example, the seed mantra for *muladhara chakra* is the sound "lam" (pronounced "lonng").

There are different ways of using mantras. The most powerful way is silent, mental repetition, but mantras can also be whispered, spoken or chanted. In each case the purpose is to "anchor" your mind and experience the vibration of the mantra throughout your physical and subtle bodies (see page 21). Traditionally, a mantra is given to you by your guru and you should neither change nor disclose it to anyone. However, in the absence of a guru, you can select a mantra and repeat it to yourself at any time, to help calm and focus your mind, as well as during meditation. When choosing a mantra there are four levels to consider: the sound of the word (or words); the meaning; the idea it embodies; and its spiritual significance. For example, words such as "love", "peace" and "harmony" are suitable mantras.

## Trataka

Trataka is an exercise in concentration that leads you naturally into a meditative state. It is also a kriya (cleansing exercise) for the eyes. Avoid trataka if you are epileptic.

To practice trataka sit in your chosen meditation position (see pages 118–19) and choose a static point or object to focus upon. This should be roughly at eye level and can be an object such as a small statue, a detail in a picture or any simple item you have to hand. You can also

*The top of a tree or the peak of a distant mountain are perfect points to focus upon during the concentration exercise trataka. The aim of trataka is to train the mind to rest upon a visual point through unblinking gaze.*

practise trataka in a natural environment where you can choose a beautiful feature of the landscape such as a tree, flower or rock or a mountain peak to focus upon. Gaze at your chosen object, keeping your eyes relaxed and steady. Don't stare or lose your point of focus – your aim is to look clearly without strain. Keep gazing without blinking until your eyes begin to water (the watering of the eyes cleanses them). When this happens, close your eyes and spend a few moments visualizing your object behind closed lids at ajna chakra (on your forehead, between your eyes; see page 25). Open your eyes again and resume gazing at your object. Repeat this opening and closing of your eyes for several minutes. Try to practice trataka for longer periods at each session. This level of concentration is excellent preparation for meditation, and when you are experienced at it, you can move seamlessly from concentrating on an object to being absorbed by it – meditation.

## Candle meditation

To practise this simple meditation technique, place a lighted candle at eye level, or slightly lower, and sit in a comfortable meditation posture. Look steadily at the

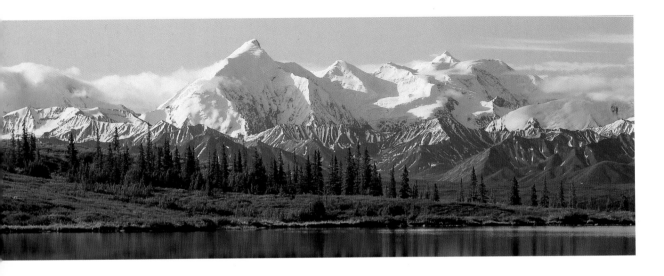

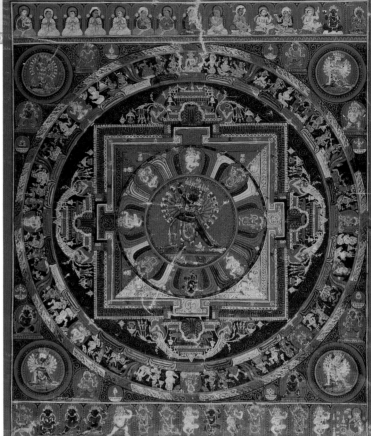

*This elaborate mandala was created in Tibet in the 15th century. In the centre, it depicts the deity Hevajra — who has 16 arms — embracing his consort Nairatmya.*

flame and calmly focus your mind upon it. Your mind may quickly wander off, but as soon as you become aware that you are distracted, try to guide yourself back to the flame and continue to gaze at it. Unlike *trataka*, you can blink whenever you need to, but if your eyes start to feel tired, close them and visualize the candle flame behind closed lids at *ajna chakra*. Don't worry if you cannot keep your mind still — with regular practice this will come more readily. A candle flame is pleasant to focus upon and has symbolic qualities associated with light and ritual, but you can practise this type of meditation with any object.

## Yantra and mandala meditation

In the same way that mantras (see page 121) are used to focus the mind through sound, *yantras* bring focus through the sense of sight. *Yantras* are two- or three-dimensional geometric representations of the levels of energy in the universe. Whether elaborate or simple in design, *yantras* usually comprise a square enclosing circles, lotus petals and triangles with a *bindu*, or seed point, at the centre.

A *mandala* is a particularly elaborate and pictorial type of *yantra* made up of and enclosed by circles (the word "*mandala*" means "circle"). The circles represent the concept of union that is at the core of yoga. *Mandalas* are commonly used in Tibetan Tantrism and usually include triangle shapes pointing both upward and downward representing Shiva and Shakti, the male and female cosmic principles. Their union within the circle represents a union of opposites — of hot and cold, sun and moon, male and female.

To begin your meditation choose a *yantra* or *mandala* (or you can use the OM symbol; see page 121) and place it at eye level so that your gaze can be steadily directed without effort. You can look at the image directly or visualize it behind closed eyes. If your eyes are open, allow them to trace the image, exploring the shape of every curve and angle and the spaces between them. Then settle your gaze in the centre of the image and absorb the shape into your mind. If your eyes become tired, continue to visualize the image behind closed eyelids.

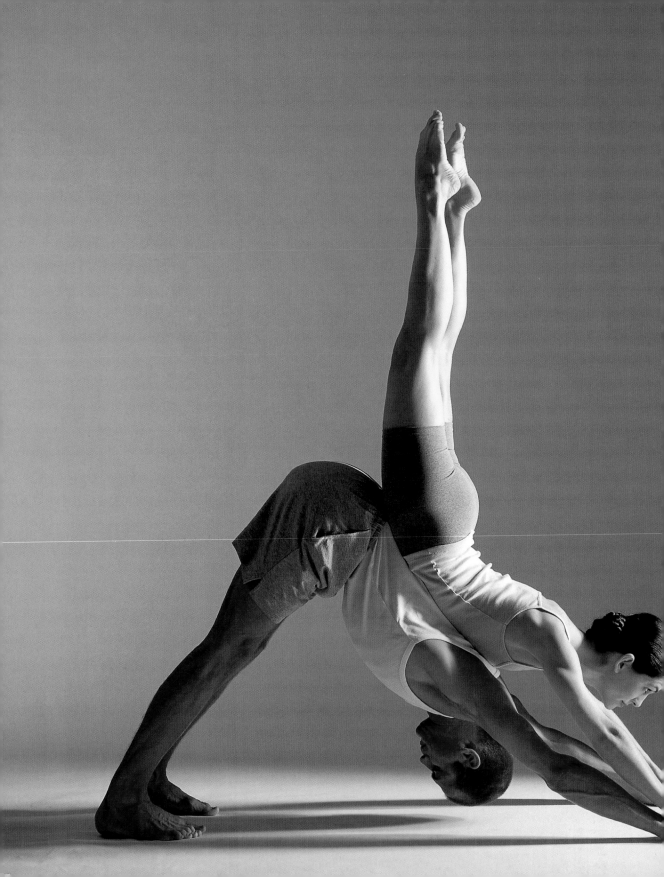

# yoga with a partner

Yoga is traditionally practised alone. Its ultimate purpose – self-realization – means that you must necessarily practise yoga by yourself, for yourself. However, there can be times when a partner is of huge benefit in terms of both providing motivation and encouragement, and offering physical support. Working with a partner enables you to learn about your body, increase the level of trust and connection between you both, and gain greater insight into the postures.

Some of the following postures are simple and gentle while others are more complex. Make sure that both of you are happy doing a posture on your own before you try the version with your partner. Be sensible about what you can attempt and be careful if one of you is significantly heavier or taller than the other – take time to find your balance. You will gain as much from the role of supporter as you will from being supported.

# the partner postures

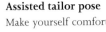

You should both be thoroughly warmed up before attempting any of these postures (with the exception of back-to-back breathing; see opposite) – start with a basic posture practice or a sequence such as sun salutation (see pages 100–101). Work closely with your partner throughout the following postures; if you are the one being supported, give your partner any essential feedback but reserve detailed discussion for later. Both of you should make slow movements – never move in to or out of a posture quickly. If something causes either of you discomfort or pain, release the posture gently.

### Assisted tailor pose
Make yourself comfortable in tailor pose (see page 74) while your partner kneels behind you. Synchronize your breathing with your partner. Your partner should place their hands on your thighs – not your knees – and gently press outward and downward on an out-breath. Continue for several breaths. Your partner should check whether the amount of pressure feels right and make adjustments accordingly.

### Forward bend
Sit on the floor, legs outstretched and feet together. Your partner stands, feet turned out. Rest your feet against the fronts of their ankles and clasp their hands or wrists. They will gently lift and stretch your arms, drawing them forward and up to lengthen your low back. Your partner should check your face and breathing for signs of strain.

Most of us find forward-bending postures challenging – working with a partner is a good way to get some assistance. It promotes correct posture and both partners will benefit from a greater understanding of the forward-bending technique.

## Back-to-back breathing

Sit back-to-back in tailor pose (see page 74), half- or full lotus (see page 75) or in a crossed-leg position. Make sure that neither of you is leaning forward or backward – you should be gently supporting each other. Use a block to sit on if you need to, but if you do, make sure that your partner sits on one too. Both place your hands on your knees or ankles or in your lap.

Once you have both settled in the posture, tune in to your own breathing pattern and concentrate on the sound of your breath. Then transfer your awareness to your back and feel your breath moving there. Feel the same movement coming from your partner and let your breathing patterns harmonize. You can stay in this position for as long as you like.

🕉 This posture is a lovely way to share some quiet time together and helps to develop acute awareness of both the breath and the back surface of the body. It is very useful if one or both of you find it difficult to maintain a sitting position on your own. This is a particularly comforting and supportive posture to do with a partner or friend if you are pregnant.

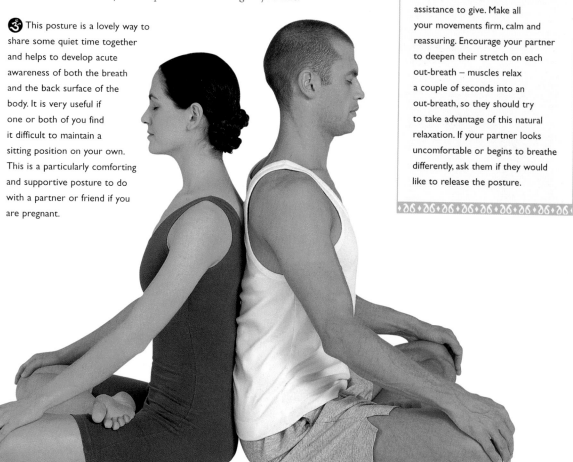

---

🕉 **GENERAL ADVICE FOR SUPPORTING PARTNERS**

When you are in a supporting role, synchronize your breathing with your partner's. Check their responses throughout the posture, giving guidance and, when necessary, asking questions so that you can judge how much assistance to give. Make all your movements firm, calm and reassuring. Encourage your partner to deepen their stretch on each out-breath – muscles relax a couple of seconds into an out-breath, so they should try to take advantage of this natural relaxation. If your partner looks uncomfortable or begins to breathe differently, ask them if they would like to release the posture.

### Back stretch

Adopt child pose (see page 68) and rest your arms on the floor in front of your head. Your partner brings the back of their hips into the back of your hips, supporting themselves with their hands on the floor. They gently roll back until outstretched on your back. They straighten their legs, relax their head and lift their arms over your head. Catch hold of your partner's wrists. Gently extend their arms forward and down.

Your partner can make this *asana* easier by bending their legs.

This stretch can elicit a strong emotional response from your partner. If this happens they should come down gently into child pose to rest.

### Double forward bend

Fold into a standing forward bend (see page 55) with your feet slightly apart, your hands on the floor for stability and your knees slightly bent. Your partner carefully steps in behind you to do the same pose. Try to touch at the hips and bring your heels as close together as possible. Take hold of your partner's ankles or shins and they should take hold of yours. Now breathe in together and both straighten your legs. On the out-breath both draw your heads toward each other's heels. Hold this position for several breaths.

In this version of a forward bend you use your partner as a stabilizing weight, or anchor, to draw yourself into a deeper bend. It works brilliantly if you are sufficiently flexible to fold forward and touch your toes, but is worth trying even if you are not.

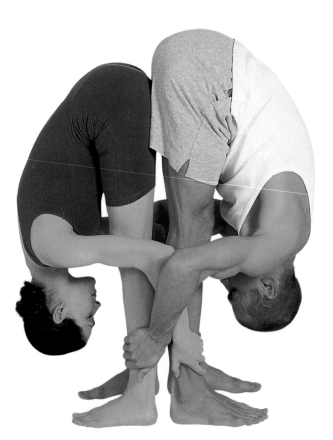

## Assisted down-facing dog

Adopt down-facing dog (see page 62). Your partner steps one foot between your hands and presses one hand in to the middle of your sacrum (back of hips). Your partner should then push firmly up and away from themselves (both hands can be placed on either side of your sacrum for more power). Release your shoulders and broaden your chest. Your partner should listen in to your breathing and encourage you to press your heels down toward the floor. (You should not move your hands closer to your feet as your partner pushes.)

🕉 This may not look very impressive but it feels great! Your understanding of down-facing dog is infinitely enhanced – working with a partner helps you to lengthen the spine, use the pelvic floor and abdominal locks (see page 107), stretch your legs and focus your mind. You really get a sense of gravity and an understanding of how this posture can prepare you for inverted postures.

## Two dogs

Adopt down-facing dog. Your partner places their feet on either side of you in line with your shoulders, then puts their hands on the floor and goes into down-facing dog. They carefully lift first one and then the other leg, placing their feet into the back of your hips (where their hands were in assisted down-facing dog, above). Their feet can be slightly turned out. They push steadily with their legs, giving you a strong stretch. They exit the pose by stepping down one foot at a time – not by jumping!

🕉 This is a powerful variation of the posture – make sure that you can stay in down-facing dog on your own for at least 10–15 breaths and have practised assisted down-facing dog posture first.

### 🕉 THE BENEFITS OF WORKING WITH A PARTNER

- Your partner can draw you more deeply into a posture using the pressure of their hands or the weight of their body. Once you are aware of how the correct posture feels you can apply this knowledge to posture practice on your own.
- Working with a partner can enhance your awareness of the breath.
- A partner is able to provide psychological support, encouragement and motivation, particularly when you lack confidence about a posture.
- Yoga with a partner encourages the development of intimacy and trust between you.
- Working with a partner can increase the incentive to practise yoga at home.

## Double triangle

Stand back-to-back with your partner with your feet wide apart. Your heels should be close to your partner's but not quite touching as you prepare for triangle (see page 56). Turn your right foot out as your partner turns their left foot out, and both breathe in and lift your arms to shoulder height. Both look down in the same direction – toward your right and their left ankles as you fold deeply in to your respective hip sockets and lengthen your sides together. You should both place your lower hands at the same point on the leg. When you feel balanced, look up and gently bring the palms of your top hands together. Stay in the pose for a few breaths, spinning the torso open toward your top hands. To come out of the position, look down, release your top hands and gently come back to standing. Repeat the posture on the other side.

🕉 The gentle touch of your connecting hands can help you both to rotate the torso fully open and stretch the upward arm.

❗ When going in and out of the posture, take care not to knock each other over!

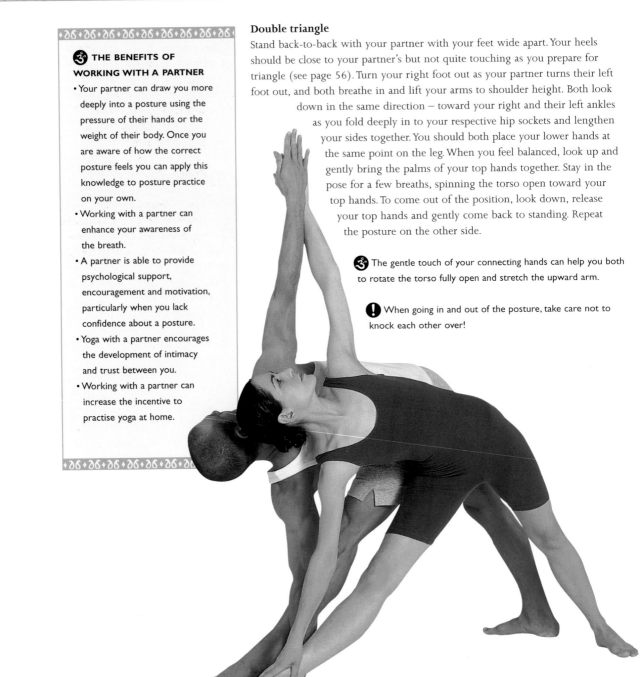

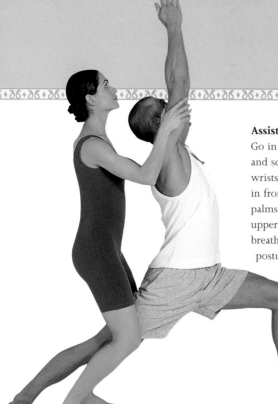

## Assisted warrior

Go in to warrior pose 1 (see page 60). Your partner steps in behind you and squeezes your back thigh between their legs. They take hold of your wrists and slowly draw your arms forward and round in a large circle – in front, down to the floor, out to the sides and back up so that your palms meet again over your head. They then transfer their grip to your upper arms – just beneath your elbows – and lift firmly. After several breaths in this position, they release their grip and step out of the posture. You return to a standing position and then repeat the pose on the other side of the body with assistance from your partner.

🕉 Your partner may not feel as though they are contributing much to this posture but you will experience a wonderful sense of freedom and space in the arms, chest, upper back, and neck. This is especially true if you usually feel tension and stiffness when you lift your arms and upper back in warrior pose.

## Squatting balance

Stand a little way apart and face each other. Hold onto each other's wrists firmly with your arms fully outstretched. Lengthen your backs and plant your feet firmly about hip-width apart. Lean slightly away from each other and start bending your knees. Come down slowly into a squatting position. Keep leaning away in order to hold the balance. Return to standing in the same way. Make your descent and ascent even, slow and steady.

🕉 This apparently simple exercise develops a sense of balance and co-ordination. It explores the possibilities of counterbalance and centres of gravity. If you and your partner are of different heights, go slowly, finding your equilibrium breath by breath.

🪷 If you find this balance easy, hold one hand with your partner rather than two (right hand to right hand and then left to left).

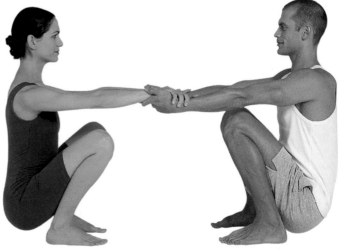

## Assisted bridge pose

Lie on your back, arms by your sides, knees bent, feet parallel (hip-width apart), and close to the hips. Tilt your pelvis upward and lift your hips off the ground as if in preparation for bridge pose (see page 77). Interlace your fingers behind your back. Draw your shoulders together. Your partner sits at your head and puts their feet against your shoulders. They put their hands underneath your upper back and draw your upper back toward them to open your chest. Your partner should steady you and themselves with their feet.

🕉 Lifting and opening the upper back and chest helps all back-bending postures by increasing the openness and flexibility of the spine.

❗ If this posture causes you any pain in the back or neck, come down slowly.

## Assisted full backbend

Lie on your back as if in preparation for the wheel (see page 82) with your feet hip-width apart, parallel and close to your body. Your partner positions their feet just behind your shoulders. Bring your arms over your head and firmly clasp your partner's ankles. Lift your hips off the floor and come in to bridge pose. Your partner reaches down and places their hands underneath your upper back. As you push up into a full backbend they draw their hands toward themselves to open and lift your chest. They may need to lean back quite a long way with their hips to hold this pose – they should bend their knees rather than their back. They may also need to adjust position depending on your flexibility. (If you feel compression in the low back, your partner is standing too close to your shoulders and you should come down while they adjust their position.) To leave the posture, they lower you to the ground, encouraging you to tuck in your chin and touch the back of your head to the floor first. Roll down the rest of your spine and do a forward bend (see page 55) to counterbalance the pose.

🕉 Don't worry about putting too much pressure on your partner's ankles – it doesn't hurt!

## Relaxation with a partner

One of the nicest things you can do for your partner at the end of a yoga practice is to help them to go in to relaxation posture (see page 89). If you feel at all nervous about working with a partner, this is also a simple and effective way to begin.

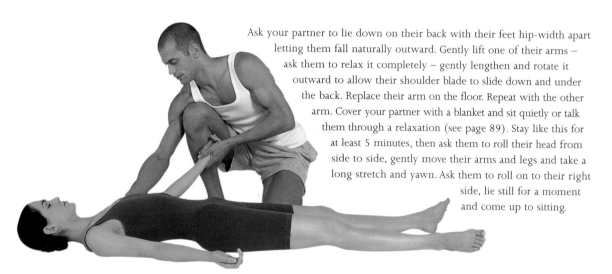

Ask your partner to lie down on their back with their feet hip-width apart letting them fall naturally outward. Gently lift one of their arms – ask them to relax it completely – gently lengthen and rotate it outward to allow their shoulder blade to slide down and under the back. Replace their arm on the floor. Repeat with the other arm. Cover your partner with a blanket and sit quietly or talk them through a relaxation (see page 89). Stay like this for at least 5 minutes, then ask them to roll their head from side to side, gently move their arms and legs and take a long stretch and yawn. Ask them to roll on to their right side, lie still for a moment and come up to sitting.

### OTHER ADJUSTMENTS FOR RELAXATION

Apart from rotating the shoulder blades back by lifting the arms, there are two other adjustments that are very helpful in this relaxation posture. If your partner's chin is lifting upward, gently place your hands on either side of their head and slightly lengthen the back of their neck. If their chin remains elevated, place a block, book or folded blanket underneath their head. The other adjustment applies to the legs. Move down to your partner's feet and lift their left leg a little way off the floor. Ask them to relax it completely so that its whole weight rests in your hands. Gently lengthen their leg away from the hip socket then lower it. Now repeat with the right leg. Make all of your movements slow, calm, firm and reassuring. Adjustments that are tentative, rough or tickly can make it difficult for your partner to relax.

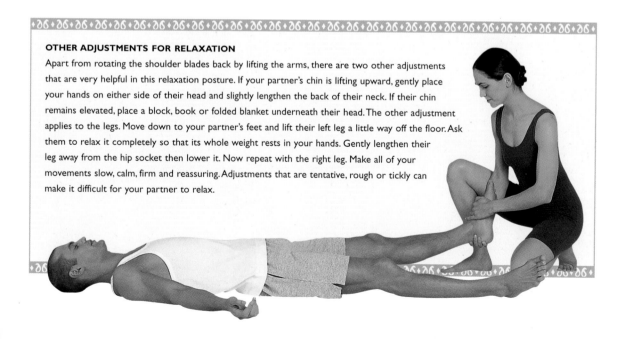

# conclusion

Wherever you are along your own personal path of yoga, I hope this book has given you encouragement and support. You will know that it is possible to practise yoga whatever your level of fitness or personal circumstances – yoga is essentially a practise for your soul, working through the medium of your body. Think of the physical benefits of yoga as profound and long-lasting side-effects of a practice that works on a very deep level.

It is said that every step along the path of yoga brings you nearer to enlightenment. Every moment spent seeking that state – whether consciously or unconsciously – is a moment well used. Even if you cease to practise yoga, you do not slip backwards as much as stand still. The *Bhagavad Gita* says that: "In this yoga, even the abortive attempt is not wasted. Nor can it produce a contrary result."

If you feel inspired to find out more about yoga, there are three main ways to do this. The first is reading. The bibliography on page 138 could serve as a starting point. It includes titles that cover the history, philosophy, physical practice and cultural significance of yoga.

The second way is learning from other people. A yoga teacher can help you to transform your practice. This does not mean that you must attend a weekly class – that may not be possible – but you could attend classes occasionally. You could also go to workshops and on courses. These are held all over the world – some last for one day or a weekend; others are short holidays that combine yoga with other activities, such as walking, painting or even windsurfing. Ashrams and retreats offer an opportunity to study yoga more seriously, perhaps under the guidance of a swami or guru. The best way to find out about all of these options is through yoga institutes (see page 139), the Internet or specialist yoga magazines.

The third and most important way to explore yoga is the simplest. Practise! Apply the skills that you already have – however basic – and you will discover more about yourself than you ever can from a mountain of books or a lifetime of classes. This is the essence of all the ancient texts; the distillation of so many minds working on these ideas over centuries. *Hathayoga Pradipika* says: "Any person, if he actively practises yoga becomes a *siddha* [adept]." The benefits of yoga are not obtained by "mere theoretical reading of the texts" or just by wearing the right clothes or by talking about yoga. "Untiring practice is the secret of success. There is no doubt about that."

What more straightforward instruction could we have?

# yoga for common ailments

| | PERIOD PAIN | MILD BACK PAIN | DIGESTIVE COMPLAINTS |
|---|---|---|---|
| RECOMMENDED *ASANAS* (POSTURES) SEE CHAPTERS 4 & 5 | Tailor pose, hero pose/reclining hero pose, child pose, knees-to-chest pose, tree pose, cow-face pose, sitting side stretch, half lotus/lotus, twist A, crow (stage 1). | Mountain pose, gentle forward bend, warrior pose (variation 2), down-facing dog, tree pose, child pose, knees-to-chest pose, hero pose (step 1), twist A, headstand (see general comments). | All forward-bending, inverted, twisting and backbending postures. |
| *ASANAS* THAT SHOULD BE AVOIDED | Plough, shoulderstand, headstand and any other inverted poses or ones that put pressure on the uterus. | Strong forward bends, backbends or twists and unsupported side-bending postures. | If your symptoms are severe, make sure your practice is gentle (for example, choose the gentle sequence on pages 96–7). |
| RECOMMENDED *PRANAYAMA* (BREATHING) EXERCISES SEE CHAPTER 6 | Alternate nostril breathing, *sitali* breath. | *Ujjayi* breath, alternate nostril breathing, *sitali* breath, extending the breath and breath retention. | All the breathing exercises in Chapter 6. |
| GENERAL COMMENTS | Remember to keep your water intake high (see pages 36–7) and cut down on caffeine. Meditation can be an excellent way to combat the symptoms of PMS – try to do a few minutes in the morning and evening. | Back pain is often a symptom of stress, which yoga can alleviate – if posture practice is too uncomfortable, try meditation or breathing back-to-back with a partner (see page 127). If you have a serious or chronic spinal injury, such as a slipped disk, you should practise yoga postures only under the guidance of a qualified yoga therapist. Only attempt a headstand if you feel confident in your technique and if headstand is not contraindicated (for example, when suffering from neck injuries). | Digestive complaints are often stress-related, so any relaxing yoga practice, such as daily meditation or the gentle sequence in Chapter 7 can be helpful. All breathing exercises are good because, as well as aiding relaxation, they help to strengthen the abdominal area. Try to follow the advice about approaches to eating in Chapter 2. Make sure, for example, that you eat your meals in a relaxed way – not in front of the television, computer screen or while reading a book. |

| INSOMNIA | UPPER BACK AND NECK AND SHOULDER TENSION | HIGH BLOOD PRESSURE | ARTHRITIS |
|---|---|---|---|
| Shoulderstand, plough, bridge pose, fish, tree pose, mountain pose (either variation), cobra, eagle pose, crescent-moon pose, any twisting postures. | Eagle pose, down-facing dog, child pose, camel pose, bridge pose, cobra, shoulderstand, plough and fish. | Corpse pose, mountain pose and hero pose. | Gentle stretching postures, such as the half-sun salutation. |
| If you are doing your practice late in the evening, avoid strong postures and focus on gentle ones to avoid overstimulation. | If tension is severe, avoid shoulderstand, plough and fish. | Avoid all inverted poses. | Avoid all postures when joints are very painful and inflamed. |
| *Ujjayi* breath, humming-bee breath, counting the breath and alternate nostril breathing. | Humming-bee breath and counting the breath. | Any gentle breathing exercise, such as alternate nostril breathing. | Any gentle breathing exercise, such as alternate nostril breathing. |
| Meditating before you go to bed at night is an excellent way to calm and balance the mind and body in preparation for sleep (unless your insomnia is caused by depression, in which case you should avoid meditation). Even if you find it hard to meditate, try to have some "quiet time" before you go to bed – no TV or radio.<br><br>As you lie in bed you may find that it helps simply to concentrate on the flow of your breath as you inhale and exhale. Try to let go of all the tension in your muscles as you do when you lie in corpse pose. | Focus your practice on complete relaxation in corpse pose. Daily meditation and breathing back-to-back with a partner (see page 127) can also help to relieve tension. | High blood pressure is a potentially serious condition. Make daily relaxation and meditation the focus of your practice and consult a yoga therapist about an *asana* practice that is specially tailored for you. | Yoga can help by stimulating blood circulation and releasing stiff joints. But make sure that you relax into *asanas* gently.<br><br>Meditation is useful in cases of rheumatoid arthritis because it balances your immune system (rheumatoid arthritis is an auto-immune disorder). |

# bibliography

Aurobindo, Sri (trans.) *The Upanishads* (Sri Aurobindo Ashram Trust, Pondicherry, India, 1996)

Bender Birch, Beryl *Beyond Power Yoga* (Simon and Schuster, London and New York, 2000)

Bouanchaud, Bernard *The Essence of Yoga, Reflections on the Yoga Sutras of Patanjali* (Rudra Press, Oregon, 1997)

Burger, Bruce *Esoteric Anatomy* (North Atlantic Books, California, 1998)

Calais-Germain, B. *Anatomy of Movement* (Eastland Press, Seattle, Washington, 1994)

Dasgupta, S.N. *Yoga Philosophy in Relation to other Systems of Indian Thought* (Motilal Barnarsidass Publishers, Delhi, India, 1996)

Desikachar, T.K.V. *The Heart of Yoga* (Inner Traditions International, New York, 1995)

Easwaran, E. (trans.) *The Upanishads* (Penguin, London, 1987/Nilgiri Press, 1987)

Eliade, Mircea *Yoga, Immortality, and Freedom* (Princeton University Press, New Jersey, 1969)

Feuerstein, G. *The Shambhala Encyclopedia of Yoga* (Shambhala, London and Boston, 1997)

Feuerstein, G. *The Yoga Tradition* (Hohm Press, California, 1998)

Hewitt, James *The Complete Yoga Book* (Rider, London, 1983)

Isherwood, C. (ed.) *Vedanta for the Western World* (Allen & Unwin, London, 1951/The Viking Press, New York, 1960)

Iyengar, B.K.S *Light on Pranayama* (Thorsons, London and New York, 1992)

Iyengar, B.K.S *Light on Yoga* (Thorsons, London, 1991/Schocken Books, New York, 1995)

Iyengar, Geeta, S. *Yoga, A Gem for Women* (Timeless Books, Washington, 1990)

Leadbeater, C.W. *The Chakras* (Quest Books, Illinois, 1987)

Mehta, Silva, Mira Mehta and Shyam Mehta *Yoga the Iyengar Way* (Dorling Kindersley, London, 1990/Knopf, Maryland, 1990)

Prabhavananda, Swami and Isherwood, Christopher (trans.) *The Bhagavad Gita* (Element Books, Shaftsbury, Dorset, 1998/New American Library, 1993)

Radhakrishnan, S. (trans.) *The Principal Upanishads* (HarperCollins, India, 1994/Humanity Books, 1992)

Saraswati, Swami *Hatha Yoga Pradipika* (Bihar School of Yoga, Bihar, India, 1985)

Satyananda Saraswati, Swami *Asana Pranayama Mudra Bandha* (Bihar School of Yoga, Bihar, India, 1966)

Schiffman, Erich *Yoga, the Spirit and Practice of Moving into Stillness* (Pocket Books, New York, 1996)

Stewart, Mary *Yoga Over 50* (Little, Brown and Co. (UK), London, 1995/Fireside Books, New York, 1994)

Vishnu-devananda, Swami *Hatha Yoga Pradipika* (Lotus, New York, 1997)

Whicher, Ian *The Integrity of the Yoga Darsana* (State University, New York, 1998)

Wood, Ernest *Seven Schools of Yoga* (Quest Books, Illinois, 1998)

Wood, Ernest *Yoga* (Penguin, London and New York, 1959)

# useful addresses

**You can contact Tara Fraser at Yoga Junction at:**

The Shiatsu Place
97–99 Seven Sisters Road
London N7 7QP
Telephone: 00 44 20 7263 3313
E-mail: info@yogajunction.com

**Other addresses:**

**In the UK**

British Wheel of Yoga
1 Hamilton Place
Boston Road
Sleaford NG34 7ES

Iyengar Yoga Institute
223A Randolph Avenue
London W9 1NL

Sivananda Yoga Vedanta Centre
51 Felsham Road
London SW15 1AZ

Viniyoga
Paul Harvey
48 Devonshire Buildings
Bath BA2 4SU

Yoga Biomedical Trust
PO Box 140
Cambridge CB4 3SY

Yoga and Health Magazine
21 Caburn Crescent
Lewes
East Sussex BN7 1NR

Yoga Therapy Centre
Royal London Homeopathic Hospital
60 Great Ormond Street
London WC1N 3HR

**In the US**

American Sanskrit Institute
73 Four Corners Road
Warwick
NY 10990

Himalayan Institute of Yoga
Science and Philosophy
RR1 Box 400,
Honesdale
PA 18431

International Association of Yoga
Therapists
209 Hillside Avenue
Milly Valley
CA 94941

Sivananda Yoga Vedanta Center
234 West 24th Street
New York
NY 10011

Yoga Journal
PO Box 469088
Escondidio
CA 92046-9088

Yoga Journal's Book and Tape Resource
2054 University Avenue
Berkeley
CA 94704-1082

**In Australia**

International Yoga Teachers
Association and Yoga for Health
Foundation
23 Morgan Street
Thornleigh
NSW 2120

**In India**

The Ramamani Iyengar Memorial Yoga
Institute
1107-B/1 Shivaji Nagar
Pune
411016

Sivananda Yoga Vedanta Centre
52 Community Centre
East of Kailash
New Delhi
110065

Vivekananda Kendra Yoga Research
Foundation
37 IV Main Road
Malleswaram
Bangalore
560003

# index

# acknowledgments

## Picture credits

The publisher would like to thank the following people, museums and photographic libraries for permission to reproduce their material. Every care has been taken to trace copyright holders. However, if we have omitted anyone, we apologise and will, if informed, make corrections in any future edition.

page 14 AKG, London/British Library; page 16 ffotograff/© Jill Ranford; page 17 AKG, London/Jean-Louis Nou; page 18 AKG, London/British Library; page 20 Images Colour Library; page 22 Images Colour Library; page 24 AKG, London/British Library; page 29 Corbis/Lindsay Hebberd; page 35 Images Colour Library; page 45 Corbis/Nik Wheeler; page 46 The Stock Market/Rob Lewine; page 48 Corbis/Nik Wheeler; page 51 Corbis/Chris Trotman; page 106 British Library; page 117 Corbis/Arne Hodalic; page 120 Corbis/Kevin R. Morris; page 122 Images Colour Library; page 123 Chester Beatty Library, Dublin.

## Models

Tara Fraser
In-Sook Chappell
Tim Cummins

## Consultant at photographic shoots

Abby Daniel

## Make-up artist

Evelynne Stoikou

## Author's acknowledgments

I would like to thank the following people:

Abby Daniel (for supervising the photo shoots and for general help, advice and support, especially running Yoga Junction while I was writing).

Sarah Macintosh (for checking the manuscript and for her continuing encouragement).

Tim Cummins and In-Sook Chappell for modelling for the photographs so beautifully.

Kesta Desmond (a dedicated student and understanding editor).

Simon Fraser for his love and support, moral and practical.

My teachers and students, past and present, from whom I have learned so much.